Cover Design/Artwork by: Line Art Graphic Design
www.lineart.net

Photography by: Richard Armas

Order this book online at www.trafford.com/07-0174
or email orders@trafford.com

Most Trafford titles are also available at major online book retailers.

Note for Librarians: A cataloguing record for this book is available from Library and Archives Canada at www.collectionscanada.ca/amicus/index-e.html

ISBN: 978-1-4251-1712-2

We at Trafford believe that it is the responsibility of us all, as both individuals and corporations, to make choices that are environmentally and socially sound. You, in turn, are supporting this responsible conduct each time you purchase a Trafford book, or make use of our publishing services. To find out how you are helping, please visit www.trafford.com/responsiblepublishing.html

Our mission is to efficiently provide the world's finest, most comprehensive book publishing service, enabling every author to experience success. To find out how to publish your book, your way, and have it available worldwide, visit us online at www.trafford.com/10510

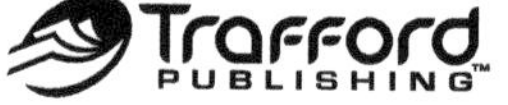

www.trafford.com

North America & international
toll-free: 1 888 232 4444 (USA & Canada)
phone: 250 383 6864 • fax: 250 383 6804
email: info@trafford.com

The United Kingdom & Europe
phone: +44 (0)1865 722 113 • local rate: 0845 230 9601
facsimile: +44 (0)1865 722 868 • email: info.uk@trafford.com

10 9 8 7 6 5 4 3 2

CONTENTS

ACKNOWLEDGEMENTS

Life is the only teacher that gives you the tests first and the lessons afterward. I'd had plenty of tests and I was qualified for a Ph.D. degree in struggling when I met C. Scott Alsop. He believes in the magic of timing and what is meant for you won't go by you.

Magic indeed! I come from a little town in Finland's farmland. Scott comes from Hollywood. I'm a nurse, Yoga teacher and author. He's a theatre, film and television writer and producer. I'm a nurturer; he's a harmonizer. I'm spontaneous; he's analytical. We both have a burning desire to improve the quality of life of people everywhere. A perfect pair, don't you think?

Scott is an inspiration to me and my two daughters, and his contribution to *A BOOMER'S HEALTH GUIDE, It's Now or Never!* has been extraordinary. For this and much more, I wish to express my deepest gratitude.

Ulla Anneli, R.N., RYT

New Year's Day, 1998 was a watershed day for me — I met Ulla. Some pretty awful life events had left me spiritually, as they say, "as low as a snake's belly." We found we had a great friend in common, the wonderful writer, humorist and author of *THE KNIGHT IN RUSTY ARMOR*, Robert Fisher. Robert "channeled" Ulla and me together, a gesture for which I will always be grateful.

In a few short months, Ulla had gently and

lovingly helped me to change my diet and other bad habits, like diet soda and saccharine, and she re-birthed and energized my battered spirit. On my birthday in February of 2002, in Montmartre, overlooking the city of Paris, Ulla consented to be my wife and, not being ones to dilly-dally, we married in May, 2002.

Since then, we have worked on many projects together, including *A BOOMER'S HEALTH GUIDE, It's Now or Never!* It's a great pleasure to help bring Ulla's message of inner peace and long, healthy life to the world.

Every day together is a gift and I am very grateful for each one.

C. Scott Alsop

FOREWORD

In my almost 25 years of practice in a major city emergency room, I can assure you I've seen it all.

I've noted that as Babyboomers pass through their 40's, 50's and 60's, more and more of them begin to appear in my emergency room. In many cases, their strokes, heart attacks, ulcers, diabetic complications, stress-related panic attacks and other serious conditions are because the years of neglect have finally caught up with them. Sometimes I even hear them say, "I knew this was going to happen."

When we know our health is at risk, either because of genetic factors or just plain neglect, why do we wait for a life-threatening event to find our motivation for positive change? Many times it's because our "force of habit" is stronger than our fear of illness and death. Sometimes it's because the information and choices available to us are confusing, contradictory and overwhelming. We need some good, common sense to help us navigate our way through the maze.

This is where Ulla Anneli, R.N., RYT comes in. I've known Ulla for about seven years now, and in that time she has had a positive and lasting effect on me and my family. Ulla's motivation is simple: she wants to help everyone reduce their stress levels and improve their health. Her knowledge is deep and varied and her approach in person and in her writing is caring, gentle, direct and encouraging.

If you're a Boomer, a pre-Boomer or a post-Boomer and you want to find a better-health-for-life program that's just right for you, *A Boomer's Health Guide, It's Now or Never*!, by Ulla Anneli, R.N., RYT is a great place to start.

Mark Rubin, M.D.

INTRODUCTION

What follows are a few of the things in my background and experience that have led me to offer this book to you and how you may use this book to potentially great advantage.

You might be asking yourself, "Who is this Ulla Anneli and what's so special about this book?" Good questions.

I have been a licensed Registered Nurse for many years. In that capacity, I have worked in hospital emergency rooms and as a charge nurse at a big city psychiatric hospital, where the focus was on drug and alcohol addiction. I've even worked as a cosmetic surgery post-op nurse. I've seen pretty much everything.

During my hospital nursing career, soul-killing stress was my constant companion. My discovery of Yoga and its amazing capacity to relieve stress literally saved my life. I am now a Registered Yoga Teacher with The Yoga Alliance, and I have taught more than 15,000 classes over 29 years.

I have guided many people to better health; people with serious conditions like MS, Lupus, Fibromyalgia and Arthritis, as well as stroke and cancer survivors. I have encountered patients and students in all phases of life, from age 3 to 106.

From the 1980's to the present, I have been seeing more and more people with Carpal Tunnel Syndrome and many other Repetitive Stress Injuries (RSI's), who have one thing in common: they all sit at computers for more than 5 hours per day.

A complete computer novice myself, I was nonetheless compelled to create software for these people, The Break™, to help prevent computer-related health problems and 3 Minute Vacations™, to relieve stress. I'm very gratified to know that individuals and businesses alike are benefiting from these products. If you're interested, I invite you to see them at my website, TakeTheBreak.com.

Along the way, I learned a very important truth: **a person's health is a daily, renewable resource, not something to use up until it's gone.** My mission in life was, is and always will be to bring this truth to as many people as possible.

This book, "A BOOMER'S HEALTH GUIDE, It's Now or Never!" is very special to me. Some 77 million strong, we Babyboomers are the group most at risk of losing our health. Just as in my private work with individuals, there is no one-size-fits-all path to take. Each person is a special being, with background, personality, genetics and problems unique to him/her.

Also, the Health Section in the bookstores is jam-packed with a huge array of diet and fitness books. If you're a Boomer and you want to commit to a new, healthy lifestyle, where do you begin? I decided to write a guide, covering several of the most serious issues Boomers are facing, offering my own advice and guidance, and leading you to solid, reliable books and websites where you can develop your own special program, according to your own special needs.

I say "It's Now or Never!" because after age 40, you can no longer rely on youth to protect you from your bad habits and self-neglect. I want to urge you to get started on your road to better health immediately and if I get my fondest wish, this guide will help you find the path that's best for you.

Ulla Anneli, R.N., RYT

1 FOREVER YOUNG

Of all the human struggles, none has been more unrelenting than man's attempts to avoid old age. No almighty kings, no heroes of Herculean strength, beautiful movie stars, fabulously rich Arab sheiks, men of knowledge and wisdom, prophets – not even saints – in fact no one has ever been able to elude the curse of old age. Yet, man never stopped trying.

Throughout the ages, people have sought ways to slow down the process of aging. Today, more than ever before, we agonize over our decaying bodies, and the "Fountain of Youth" cannot be had for the asking, not even for all the gold in the world. Here's the good news: we can delay our aging process and, in some cases, actually reverse our premature aging.

Thanks to modern technology, we have at our disposal everything from cosmetic surgery to promising anti-aging techniques, theories, drugs, nutrients and cosmetics. In the quest for youth, there are many options. There is, however, one area of vital research that is left unacknowledged and that is the potent capacity of the mind.

As much as 90% of the human brain lies dormant. If we were able to use only ten percent more of our brains, we would all be more intelligent. The question is this: how do we activate the brain to induce it to heal our bodies and keep them from aging, decaying, and even prematurely dying? The answer lies in our thoughts.

Thoughts of fear, pain, grief and hatred can create in us the look and feeling of old age, in spite of our chronological age. By contrast, thoughts of self-confidence, health, joy and love cause us to radiate the look and feeling of youth, again in spite of our chronological age. Aging is inevitable – growing old is not!

Whatever you think, believe and feel will most likely become your reality. Study people you know who seem so much older than their years. Invariably, you will find them to be negative, fearful, closed-minded and humorless. Likewise, you will find that people who seem younger than their years are positive, confident, open-minded and quick to smile and laugh. Your personality and your way of thinking, feeling and dealing with life's roller coaster of joy and pain are not genetic – they are learned.

The same way a brand new computer is programmed, so is the human brain. The experiences and influences of all the events of your life and how you perceive them make you who you are.

The problem is often that children and young adults don't have the experience and wisdom to analyze information as it comes in and to separate useful from useless, helpful from hurtful, and to make the right choices. Instead, all the information pours in, all the thoughts and ideas, the influences from every source and direction and there it all stays, unsorted and even unrecognized.

Some children and young people are truly blessed to have parents who are centered, positive, confident and skilled at managing life's stress. Children learn subliminally by watching and then incorporating what they learn into their own personality and attitudes.

Unfortunately, the opposite is often true. Children whose parents are scattered, negative, fearful and poor managers of stress learn and incorporate those behaviors too.

So, in adulthood, many of us come to a point when we become motivated and determined to make positive changes in our way of thinking and improve our lives. That very decision automatically opens in our brains a new pathway to information, ideas and positive change.

Every time you accept a thought that is greater than your norm, that thought stimulates your brain into new, purposeful use. This automatically stimulates other areas of the brain for more thought, information and reasoning. This desire for new thought stimulates your pituitary gland and a wonderful process begins.

The pituitary is an oval endocrine gland attached to the base of the vertebrate brain, the secretions of which control the other endocrine glands and influence growth, metabolism and maturation. The hormone flow from the pituitary goes deep into the brain mass and stimulates the pineal gland. From the pineal, it travels to and stimulates the thymus gland. In most people, the thymus is usually the size of a pea. It should be the size of a peach! The thymus gland starts to shrink at puberty. For us to retard aging, the thymus must be stimulated through the pineal. Positive emotions activate and strengthen this gland and, in this, could very well lie the secret of immortality

.

There has been some speculation from researchers

that a serum could be developed that could stimulate the pituitary gland and maintain our youth, vitality and health indefinitely. Naturally, this would signal the end for many major industries which thrive on illness and aging, so it's safe to assume we won't be seeing this "magic potion" any time soon. We'll just have to move our hormones and cancel the death message in our pituitaries ourselves!

We start the process by bringing in new and exciting thoughts and waking up our minds. We must work on developing the consciousness of a happy child. Happy kids view life with a sense of simplicity and expectancy. They explore life with open hearts and minds and the unknown is only a curiosity, not something to fear. They love themselves, as well they should. They live in the moment.

To acquire this childlike attitude, practice visualizing a young, happy child within you just before you fall asleep each night. Suggest to your subconscious mind, something like: "There is inside of me a spiritual, joyful being – ever young, ever beautiful, ever healthy, ever loving. This Divine and powerful child influences every aspect of my being in a positive way. And my Divine chemist is making all the repairs my body needs, while I sleep." When you awaken, take a moment to visualize this amazing inner child and your infallible chemist. If you like, you can even say, "Good morning."

These repeated affirmations are powerful and they can bring positive change and even complete transformation. Your skin will appear healthier and a renewed spirit of youth will appear in your step, your attitude and your outlook. Don't believe me? Try it!

Did you ever hear the expression, "a smile is the best facelift?" Learn to smile in the sweet way of a child. A child's smile comes from the soul. Open your soul to happy thoughts and, when they come, show them on your face. In each genuine smile there is eternal youth.

Learn to thrill yourself. When you see something beautiful, don't just look – feel. When positive ideas and emotions hit you, don't just feel them, say, "Wow!" From this will come new enthusiasm and youthful energy.

Balance is critical to a happy, healthy, youthful life. Strive to balance your diet, exercise, work, relationships, thoughts and attitudes. A youthful attitude can add years to your life and, at the same time, can add life to your years.

Here are a few simple rules to live by:

1. Avoid aggravation by not taking life too seriously. Apply your sense of humor to life's everyday absurdities and you'll find yourself laughing more than crying.

2. Don't agonize over failures. You may have learned to do that in your childhood and it may well lead you to low self-esteem. Failure can teach humility. Humility can teach self-forgiveness. Self-forgiveness is a gateway to wisdom.

3. Work on being patient. Things just naturally happen in their own time and for the patient, positive person, when that time comes, good

things are unstoppable. Keep in mind that impatience and restlessness lead to dissatisfaction and unhappiness. Patience and inner peace go hand in hand.

4. Serve others. You will often receive joy and personally benefit from simple, selfless acts of generosity, often more than the persons receiving them will.

But there's more. Lots more. Our minds are the ultimate anti-aging power we all possess, so please open your mind to these concepts. Some are new and challenging. Others are old, almost timeless.

PROPER CARE AND FEEDING OF YOUR BRAIN

Let's take a few moments and talk about your brain.

You've probably lived all your years 'til now without giving much thought to this incredible organ of yours. Every heartbeat, every breath, every thought — literally every step you've taken so far has begun in your brain.

The quality of your "Golden Years" depends in large part on the health and efficiency of your brain. Have you taken good care of it? Do you know how?

Like most of your muscles, if you use your brain and don't abuse it, it will stay fit and serve you well for a long time. Also like your muscles, if don't give your brain the fuel and exercise it needs, it will atrophy.

So, while you're developing your own personal health and fitness program for the rest of your body, please pay special attention to your brain.

BRAIN FOODS

Omega 3 fatty acids, fish (fresh and wild if you can get it), walnuts and Siberian Ginseng all offer terrific nutrition for your brain. Also, Coenzyme Q10, which some nutritionists call "the miracle vitamin of the 1990's", helps increase energy at the cellular level.

The old joke goes: a man says, "Doc, I'm having problems with my memory." Doc asks, "How long have you had this problem?" The man asks, "What problem?"

The fact is, as you age, you may notice a tendency to forget your keys or glasses. You may also notice that you remember the name of the doctor you had 30 years ago but you can't remember the name of the one you just saw last week.

Maybe you've had the experience of blanking on a name you know well and you begin a search through your memory: "He went to Yale, his first wife was Florence, they had three kids, Bill, Johnny and Marge" — until you say, "Aw, the heck with it!" Then, much later, without any thought at all, boom! — there's the name. But now you can't remember why you needed it!

These "Senior Moments", as they're so aptly called, are normal. Your synapses and their neurotransmitters are firing a little slower, true, but you might also be stressed out or getting a little worried about your memory, which actually interferes with the memory process. When you're always in a hurry or multi-tasking too much, it's difficult to focus your brain on one specific thought or activity. Unresolved anger and lack of quality sleep tend to retard brain function. Excessive use of alcohol and drugs, prescription or otherwise, destroy brain cells — and brain cells, for all intents and purposes, don't re-generate.

If you've lived 50 years or more, think of all the information that's been stored in your memory! If your brain were a computer, you would have changed your hard drive several times by now.

Consider taking some of these nutrients that support your memory function: Vitamins B-12, E and C, Folic Acid, Copper, Zinc, Calcium, Magnesium, Boron, Lecithin and DHEA. Look for a high-quality supplement which targets the brain's memory function. Ginkgo Biloba's stimulating effect has shown to be more effective in people with declining brain power than others.

According to Fernando Gómez-Pinilla, Ph.D, a professor of Neurology at UCLA, those who are suffering from serious conditions, such as Alzheimer's, Dementia and Cerebral Insufficiency, have the most to gain from brain nutrition and exercise.

BRAIN EXERCISE

Physical activity increases blood flow to your brain and helps control blood pressure. A brisk 30-minute walk, swimming, hiking or gardening will do the trick, as long as it's mildly aerobic. Before you start any new regimen, check with your doctor first, please.

I'll bet you've heard the term "mental gymnastics." Well, I think it's a good thing to challenge your brain with new thoughts and concepts. Do crossword or jigsaw puzzles or Sudoku. Take an adult education class in something that interests you or join a discussion group or a book club. Your brain may not be tired, it might just be bored!

Make these things habitual or, as I like to say, "positive addictions".

LOVING YOU

Everything positive, even staying young, starts with self-love. Self-love has little to do with how much others love you. When you love and respect yourself, all things are possible.

First, you have to accept and be accountable for all the not-so-good choices you've made so far and the things you've done you're not proud of.

Next, forgive yourself. Sometimes it's much easier said than done, but critical nonetheless, so work on it. Apologize, make amends, do what it takes to put these things behind you.

Now, remember all the good you've brought to yourself, your family and the world – and feel good about it. All these things make you worthy of self-love. Feel it. Believe it.

CHANGE UNLOVING TO LOVING

The power of love can change your destiny. A change in your attitude can change your life.

Your subconscious mind has no sense of humor.

Everything you think and say to others is recorded in your subconscious. Every thought you have, even in your most private moments, is recorded too.

"I guess it's just old age sneaking up on me," you might say in jest. "My memory isn't what it used to be." Beware -- your subconscious mind is listening and taking notes. When you hear yourself sending negative messages about yourself outward and inward, stop! Change that bad thought into a good one, in mid-sentence if you can.

Break up the negative thought patterns which have become habit, like complaining, holding on to anger too long, self-doubt, self-loathing. Find ways of expressing out loud your appreciation and love for the smallest things in life, like a beautiful day, the smell of fresh flowers or someone's smile that made you feel better. More importantly, express your love and appreciation for the big things in life. When you begin to make a point of expressing positive emotions, you will immediately feel a difference in you, all the way down to the cellular level. You'll smile more, laugh more, hug more and smiles, laughter and hugs will come back to you.

Did you ever feel bad when you hurt someone, even if you thought he/she deserved it for hurting you first? On the other hand, was it a relief when you apologized for bad behavior? Did you ever feel a weight lifted off you when you forgave someone? That weight is your conscience, your knowledge of right and wrong, weighing on your subconscious mind. If you don't make a regular conscious effort to be pro-actively accountable, that weight can become unbearable. Express your love by forgiving and forgetting all the thousands of slights you may have suffered over your lifetime. It's not easy, but it's definitely anti-aging!

AFFIRMATIONS

What you think about, you bring about! Decide what you want. Be specific and open to receiving the highest good. See, feel and be ready to experience your brightest dreams of health and youth. Reject what you don't want to manifest in your body. Continue to condition your mind toward beauty, energy, vitality and health.

Many people have not even heard of or considered the concept of affirmation. Others find it laughable. But, remember, your subconscious is listening. All you're doing is programming it with a torrent of positive thoughts. Your subconscious, like the genie in the lamp, hears and obeys.

Affirmations are specific to each individual's needs. You will create your own accordingly. Here are a few examples:

Health -- "I am now radiantly healthy and whole."
Youth -- "I am growing younger with each breath I take.
Rejuvenation – "My body is throwing off the shackles of old age."

Mental or oral repetition must be accompanied by genuine emotion. Make sure your motivation is pure. Look for results in about twenty one days!

* *

Recommended Reading & Websites

Chasing Life: New Discoveries In The Search For Immortality To Help You Age Less Today, Sanjay Gupta, M.D., Warner Wellness, 2007, available on Amazon. Com

Naomi's Guide To Aging Gratefully: Facts, Myths And Good News For Boomers, Naomi Judd, Simon & Schuster, 2007, available on Amazon.com

Ageless: The Naked Truth About Bioidentical Hormones, Suzanne Somers, Crown, 2006

The RealAge® Makeover: Take Years Off Your Looks And Add Them To Your Life, Michael F. Roizen, M.D., HarperCollins, 2004, 2005, available on Amazon.com

Grow Younger, Live Longer, Deepak Chopra, Three Rivers Press, 2001, available on Amazon.com

Get Healthy Now!: A Complete Guide To Prevention, Treatment and Healthy Living, Gary Null, Seven Stories Press, 2006, available on Amazon.com

Healthy Aging: A Lifelong Guide To Your Well-Being, Andrew Weil, 2007, available on Amazon.com

Keep Your Brain Young: The Complete Guide To Physical And Emotional Health And Longevity, Guy M. McKhann and Marilyn Albert, John Wiley & Sons, 2002, available on Amazon.com

2 THE BREATH OF LIFE

Breath is the essence of life.

Many of us suffocate in stages due to life-long patterns of improper breathing. On the physical level, breathing supports the metabolism of every cell in the body. On a more subtle level, it acts like a bridge between the body and the mind. When this body/mind connection becomes weak and distorted, the whole system struggles to regain its equilibrium. Breathing can produce illness or vibrant health, depending on how it's used.

Most of the time, we are not even aware of our breathing. It is automatic. We take it for granted until something goes wrong, and then we realize how marvelous a mechanism we are equipped with. Surely, you have noticed how your emotions affect the flow of your breath. A sudden, fearful reaction will result in shallow, rapid breathing; while a quick, gasping breath signals we are about to cry. On the other hand, when we are relaxed, our breathing is deep and slow. You will see how we can use this relationship to calm the mind and reduce stress by regulating our breathing.

In addition to emotional stress, there are other factors which decrease our breathing efficiency and limit our feeling of wellness. Breathing through the mouth makes the mouth dry, which can lead to tooth decay. Air drawn in through the mouth is not warmed by the nasal passages and bypasses the natural filtering of nasal hairs and mucus membranes, which in turn may lead to respiratory and throat infections.

So, healthy breathing is done through the nose with proper posture and periodic "breaks" for deep breathing.

I'm constantly amazed at how many people have never even considered the possibility of conscious breathing. "I know how to breathe", they say, "I've been doing it all my life!" What they mean is that they've always left it up to their autonomic nervous systems. Yoga breathing has been around for thousands of years and most people know absolutely nothing about it.

You can breathe to energize, to relax, to calm, to focus, to concentrate. And you can breathe for health and rejuvenation.

You will be astonished by the benefits you can achieve by using the special breathing techniques outlined below.

DEEP BREATHING

In Yoga, *Prana* is known as the "vital force". It is the subtle life energy inherent in the air we breathe, the food and water we consume and the sunlight that supports life on Earth. Science has identified many of the nourishing elements in food, such as vitamins and minerals, but it is well-known that these substances alone cannot support life. Likewise, we have discovered that oxygen is the primary life supporting element in the air we breathe, but no living thing can be supported by oxygen alone. Even sunlight has important elements which science as yet has not been able to identify and measure. Life-force, then, can be said to be that essential energy we receive from the ethereal levels of our environment. According to the ancients, the life force is primarily brought in through the breath. In Yoga, the techniques for enhancing this flow are called *Pranayama*.

These exercises should be learned and performed gradually and carefully to develop the body's tolerance to the increased energy and cleansing effects they bring.

THREE-PART BREATH

Most of us take shallow breaths, using only the upper chest. Even our so-called deep-breathing is limited to the chest area by raising and lowering the shoulders. Anyone who has played a wind instrument, or has acted or sung professionally, knows that a much greater volume of air can be taken in by using the muscles of the abdomen. The three-part technique combines this diaphragmatic breathing with intercostals (mid-chest) and clavicular (upper chest) breathing. Here's how it works:

Choose a comfortable seated position, keeping the spine straight and relaxed.

1. Place the palms of your hands on your abdomen with the fingers lightly touching to check the movement of the diaphragm and stomach muscles. Begin to inhale, and let your abdominal muscles relax and expand. This allows the air to fill the deepest part of your lungs. You will notice that your fingers will part slightly as your stomach moves outward.

2. Continue to inhale, filling your mid-chest, feeling how your ribcage expands.

3. Complete your inhalation, completely filling your lungs to the top. You'll feel your collar bones gently rising.

4. Now, begin to exhale slowly, first from your upper chest.

5. Continue your exhale from your mid-chest, feeling your ribcage relaxing.

6. Finally, exhale from the bottom of your lungs, tightening your abdominal muscles to force out the last bit of air.

7. Now, relax your stomach muscles and another inhalation begins.

The difference between deep, rhythmic, conscious breathing and hyperventilation is in the exhale. When we hyperventilate, we take deep breaths but only are able to manage shallow exhalation. The result is over-oxygenation which leads to light-headedness, dizziness and even fainting.

In deep, conscious breathing, we pay equal attention to the exhalation. At the end of our inhalation, oxygen is exchanged for carbon dioxide in the lungs and the bloodstream carries the oxygen literally to every cell in our bodies. The exhalation rids us of the depleted air in the form of carbon dioxide, so it is crucial that the exhalation be as complete as the inhalation.

If you experience light-headedness when you are practicing this technique, pay more attention to your exhalation and make sure each one is complete.

By establishing a routine of at least five minutes per day, you will greatly increase the oxygenation of your blood, which will help your entire system. The average person at rest inhales only about 1,500 cubic centimeters of air per breath. The three-part technique increases your air intake up to about 3600 cubic centimeters and maintains proper elasticity of the lungs. This is especially important as we grow older because increased oxygen to the cells slows the aging process and promotes good health.

Keep in mind that shallow breathing doesn't exchange the air in the deepest part of the lungs. The carbon dioxide-heavy stale air can make us feel sluggish at the very least and can even lead to respiratory infections.

There are several other important benefits you receive from deep breathing. It gives your internal organs a gentle, kneading massage. It induces relaxation, calms the nervous system and balances the right and left sides of your brain. Ridding yourself of excess carbon dioxide and other metabolic waste helps put your body into a harmonious state. This clears your mind, stabilizes your blood pressure, freshens your skin and improves your memory and concentration. Don't believe me? Give it a try!

ENERGY BREATH

This technique is perfect for the so-called "4 o'clock slump" at the office, or any time you need to wake up and focus.

It should only be done with an empty stomach, say two hours after eating. Once again, choose a comfortable seated position, preferably cross-legged. Sit up straight and relax your shoulders.

1. Begin with a deep inhalation, allowing your stomach and abdomen to expand outward, drawing the air into the deepest part of your lungs, just like the first stage of the three part breath.

2. Quickly contract the muscles of your stomach and abdomen inward, forcing the air sharply out through your nostrils, almost like a sneeze.

3. This forceful exhalation is followed right away by a rapid inhalation as in Step 1. Remember to expand your stomach and abdomen outward again.

4. Repeat this technique 6 to 10 times, using your stomach and abdominal muscles like a "pump", concentrating on maintaining the breath at the diaphragm and below. If you do more than one round of Energy Breath, it's best to take a few normal breaths in between rounds.

Benefits include warming and energizing the body, clearing and focusing the mind, preventing lung congestion and improving digestion. Try it in the morning just after awakening; you'll love it.

BELLOWS BREATH

This technique is done like the Energy Breath, except the inhalation is much more quick and vigorous, matching the exhale. If you feel light-headed at any time, please stop and breathe normally for a few minutes. When you begin again, make sure that you are exhaling completely.

1. In the beginning, until you become accustomed to this technique, it helps to place your hands on your abdomen with your fingertips touching. Start with a full breath as before, allowing your stomach and abdominal muscles to expand and filling your lower lungs completely.

2. Contract your abdominal muscles sharply, as in Energy Breath, forcing the air out through your nose. If you like, you can push lightly on your abdomen to assist the exhalation. Once this exhalation becomes normal, you need only to sit up straight with your shoulders relaxed.

3. Inhale deeply as before, allowing your stomach and abdominal muscles to relax and filling your lower lungs. This is one round.

Begin with 10 to 12 rounds of Bellows Breath, ending each round with a deep exhalation. If you do more than one round, take a few normal breaths between rounds. Be sure to pay special attention to your exhalations, making sure they are complete.

Pranayama, the science of breath, is much more than just deep and energizing breathing. Its aim is to enable you to actually control the life force within your body and mind. Remember that *prana* is a subtle form of energy that supports, purifies and detoxifies every cell of your body. Remember, breath is the essence of life. These techniques, done regularly and correctly, are life extending.

CALMING BREATH

When you practice this simple technique, you will be amazed at how it actually alters your mental state as it balances and strengthens your nervous system. It's perfect when you're upset, angry, nervous or just plain stressed-out. If you learn and use only one of these techniques, make it Calming Breath!

1. Sit in a chair or in a comfortable cross-legged position, with your back straight and your shoulders relaxed. Make your right hand into a fist and hold it in front of your face. Release your thumb like you're making the "thumbs up" sign. Now straighten your ring and pinky fingers, extending them forward. Close your eyes.

   Inhale deeply to the top of your lungs, as in the Three Part Breath. Using your thumb, close off your right nostril and slowly exhale through your left nostril. Now inhale deeply through your left nostril. When you have a full breath, release your thumb, close off your left nostril with your ring finger and pinky and exhale slowly through your right nostril. Now inhale deeply through your right nostril until you have a full breath. This is one round of the Calming Breath.

2. Now use your thumb again to close off your right nostril and exhale through your left as before. Then it's inhale left, switch fingers, exhale right, inhale right, switch fingers, exhale left, inhale left, switch fingers, exhale right.

3. To begin, three or four rounds are sufficient, just be sure to finish by exhaling completely through your right nostril.

4. Now, return to your normal breathing and sit quietly for a few moments, listening to your breath and feeling it moving in and out.

This powerful technique can be practiced anywhere, any time to relax and center your mind and body. Begin with a minute or less and gradually increase to 5 minutes. If dizziness or discomfort occurs, stop and return to your normal breathing, paying special attention to your exhalations.

Also, if you suffer from insomnia, sinus problems and headaches, you will find this technique very helpful. It is now part of many stress management programs in businesses and hospitals. When our daily stresses cause us to go against the natural forces, we lose energy. That is why just a few minutes of relaxation and inner peace during the day can restore energy and even help us to recover from illness and long term emotional stress.

All in all, the quality of your life depends on the energy you have to give to it. Your breathing plays a critical role in building and maintaining energy levels. Conscious breathing can literally change your life, so start your practice today!

* *

Recommended Reading & Websites

Autobiography Of A Yogi, Paramhansa Yogananda, Philosophical Library, 1946, 2006, available on Amazon.com

Anatomy Of Hatha Yoga: A Manual for Students, Teachers and Practitioners, H. David Coulter, Body and Breath, Inc., 2001, available on Amazon.com

Yoga Over 50: The Way To Vitality, Health, and Energy In The Prime Of Life, Mary Stewart, Fireside/Simon & Schuster, 1994, available on Amazon.com

The New Yoga For People Over 50: A Comprehensive Guide For Midlife and Older Beginners, Suza Francina, HCI, 1997, available on Amazon.com

3 MEDITATION – HAPPINESS IN SOLITUDE

In our crowded and confrontational world, our need for refuge and self-centering is becoming increasingly important. Noisy, bustling supermarkets, shopping malls, doctor appointments, bumper-to-bumper traffic, even a boisterous household can make our world shrink until it feels like we're living in a matchbox. One escape is to seek the company of others, the so-called "security in numbers". There is another place to go. It's a peaceful place, a place where you can be alone but never be lonely, a place that is each person's personal sanctuary — it's called "within."

We all could use some slowing down for a little self-reflection. Health clubs work out our physical bodies and places of worship tend to our spiritual needs, but where do we find a quiet place where we can find some peace of mind? Within.

For the practical purposes of health and rejuvenation, meditation is an ancient routine for focus and calming the mind. How ancient? Thousands of years. Does it work? You bet. Will it work for you? Try it and see.

Think of your mind as a radio, rapidly and randomly switching from station to station. If it could stay on the good stations longer, life would be better. The human mind is an insatiable pleasure-seeker, thriving on worldly enjoyments of all kinds, big and small. Your mind has been trained that all pleasure is on the outside. If you've never asked your mind to look within, it will never go where it has never been. When your mind discovers pleasure and enjoyment within, it will want to go back again and again.

Every activity we perform in life is balanced by another activity or by inactivity. We balance work with play or rest or both. Without this balance we can't function. Balance is essential to optimum performance. Just as the race car mechanic tunes up the car's engine, so do we have to "tune up" our minds. This doesn't mean putting more information in, it means cleaning out negative and useless thoughts which block harmony and insight. The meditative state provides a much deeper relaxation than sleep does. 15 to 20 minutes of meditation slows the heartbeat and oxygen consumption drops by as much as 20%. This is comparable to an entire night of sleep. Why wouldn't a person want to meditate?

To meditate, you don't have to create any special state of mind. You let go of the "normal" turmoil and noise in your mind and reveal the peace that is always there within you. The natural condition of the mind is to be at peace. All the circumstances, expectations, desires, obsessions, dislikes, guilt, fear, et cetera, disturb that natural peaceful state. Meditation, then, is the practice of removing your mind's focus from everything that is not its true quiet, peaceful nature.

So, for those of you who have never tried meditation before, allow me to offer you a brief but effective beginning meditation.

First, choose a quiet place. Sit on the floor or in a chair and begin by staring at a candle in front of you. The flame of the candle has a powerful vibration which helps to still the mind. When your eyes start watering or blinking, close them and try to see the flame in your mind's eye. If at first you aren't successful, please don't give up — most do in the beginning. What is important at this stage is to keep trying, until you capture the flame.

When you have the flame in sight of your mind's eye, send the light to your heart, to any part of your body or to a person. How? It's personal. Use your thought and imagination. For example, imagine your heart or a loved one surrounded by beautiful, gentle, healing light and see how long you can hold that vision. Sit quietly afterward and reflect on your experience.

Don't be discouraged if dramatic results are not obtained immediately. Meditation is a discipline which "trains" the mind. It takes time and practice.

Most people find that they go through three stages. The first is ***focusing*** — simply developing the ability to bring your attention to one chosen object or word. Most meditation techniques begin by ***focusing on the rhythm of the breath***.

The second stage is ***concentration***, in which you are able to maintain uninterrupted attention on one object for an extended period of time.

The third stage is ***meditation***. Here, even the awareness of breathing is transcended and you begin to enjoy a sense of equilibrium, a feeling that everything is just right. Don't rush yourself at this point — passively observe your thoughts going by and do nothing to stop the parade.

Meditation isn't done by force or strain but by

practice. For most beginners just sitting down with the purpose of meditating seems difficult at first. The untrained mind is like an over-active child, restless and rambunctious and hard to rein in. Thoughts ricochet around, and every time the body moves, the mind wanders. That's why preparation is important. This is where ***mantra*** is used. This is a word or group of words that carry special meaning for you, which are repeated aloud, or silently in your mind, in order to help "carry" you to deeper levels of awareness.

Different systems of meditation use different *mantras*. For example, prayer can be a form of meditation. In your research, find a system of meditation which appeals to you and a *mantra* that holds important significance for you.

Always come out of meditation slowly, with the resolve to carry the quietness within you throughout the day.

No matter which system of meditation you choose, here are a few guidelines to get you started:

1. Establish a routine. Put aside at least 10 – 15 minutes each day for the practice of your meditation technique. The best times are early morning and evenings just before bed.

2. Designate an area in your home which can be regarded as your special sanctuary, where you feel comfortable and at ease. After a while, the mental association with your sanctuary will be one of harmony and serenity. This will help you relax and lead you to a meditative state of mind.

3. Start with breathing techniques. Especially helpful are the Three-part Breath and the Calming Breath discussed in the previous chapter.

4. Avoid the so-called "pitfalls of progress." As you master the technique of meditation, your mind will be brought to a state of quietness that lies just below your conscious awareness. That means no anxiety, fear, depression, — just a level of pure awareness. This taps into a wide world of intuitive knowledge which can now present itself to your conscious mind. At first, this will seem to you like a major breakthrough and it can be a tremendous factor in problem-solving — but you must eventually move beyond this level. You aren't in meditation, after all, to work out logistical problems. Your ultimate goal is a realm that transcends all thoughts. This is where the "pitfalls of progress" come in. Different levels of meditation can be quite seductive and it is important to realize that as long as you're dealing with thoughts, words, judgments and illusions, you are still engaging with your conditioned mind. The greatest benefit is found in unconscious awareness but that requires letting go of even your most profound ideas and brainstorms. Easier said than done.

No matter what level you attain, you will find that meditation is a fantastic practice which can have a profound effect on how you think, feel, react — even how you look. I have seen a spark of youth in the eyes of older people who have meditated for many years. Their skin has less wrinkles and their attitude toward life is calm and bright. It's because they are less likely to be caught up in the everyday dramas and dilemmas life assails us with.

Several hospital studies have reported that people who meditate on a regular basis don't suffer from as much degenerative disease, such as heart attack, stroke, high blood pressure, diabetes and even some cancer. The message is: ***don't medicate — learn to meditate!***

It is said that in prayer we speak to God and that in meditation God speaks to us. I hope, if you haven't done so already, that you will explore this wonderful ancient practice. It will serve you well.

* *

Recommended Reading & Websites

For beginners:

8 Minute Meditation/Quiet Your Mind, Change Your Life, Victor Davich, 2004, Perigee Books – available on Amazon.com

Meditation For Dummies, Stephan Bodian, 2006, Wiley Books – available on Amazon.com

Guided Mindfulness, John Kabat-Zinn, 2005, Audio Book, available on Amazon.com

Wherever You Go, There You Are: Mindfulness Meditation In Everyday Life, John Kabat-Zinn, 2005, available on Amazon.com

A Gradual Awakening, Stephen Levine, Anchor Books, 1989, 1993, available on Amazon.com

www.InsightMeditation.com

TakeTheBreak.com, 3 Minute Vacations™, brief video meditations on your computer

4 NUTRITION – YOU REALLY ARE WHAT YOU EAT!

No two subjects cause more disagreement among the "experts" than do DIET and LONGEVITY. Bookstore shelves are crammed full of books and studies, myriads of infomercials trumpet the latest fads and we're left with enough conflicting advice on these subjects to boggle our minds.

I don't want to add to this dilemma so I will simply offer you some helpful hints that will guide you toward finding out what's best for you.

If it's a "diet" you're seeking, sorry, you won't find it here. Most people are aware that diets are quick-fixes that lead to long-term disappointments. Some are actually dangerous to your health.

If healthy weight loss is your goal, you must first face this one very important reality: *you didn't get fat overnight so you won't get skinny overnight either!*

Permanent lifestyle changes are the answer. When you cut out or replace the things you're eating that pack on the pounds, you'll lose the pounds. The art is in creating your new eating habits so that you're well-nourished, with plenty of energy, without feelings of being deprived. Some will benefit greatly by understanding their own personal psychology of *why* they eat, what they eat and when they eat.

Much popular dietary advice belongs under the category of "fad". Artful marketing has made it almost impossible for the average person to tell the crucial difference between fact and fad. My best recommendation is for you to find a first-rate nutritionist, well-trained and experienced in his/her field. Also, when you make changes, introduce them gradually so your body and mind have time to adjust. Remember that a balanced mind is just as important as a balanced diet. Don't drive yourself crazy with radical changes, guilt and self-loathing — be gentle with yourself, change slowly but surely and congratulate yourself for each little step you take toward optimum nutrition.

Answer these questions honestly and you'll have some good clues as to where to begin:

Do you overeat because something's eating you?

Does your mood determine what you eat?

Do you eat more than you need to satisfy your appetite?

Do you "wolf" your food with minimal chewing?

Do you eat before bed and, if so, what?

What you eat and how you eat affect your entire being. You may eat large meals without getting the nutrients you need. If you eat too many sugars and carbohydrates, your mood may swing dramatically as your blood glucose level rises and falls. It's perfectly possible to be overweight and be anemic and malnourished. Make positive changes in your eating habits and it will change your life. Make those changes as delicious as they are nutritious and they will last for the rest of your life.

Here are four principles to consider:

PRINCIPLE ONE: VARIETY

Whether you're an omnivore, one who eats every type of food, or a vegetarian or vegan, variety is an important key. In every category of food you eat, strive for variety. For example, when you eat a wide variety of fruits, vegetables, grains and proteins, you'll have three important advantages: you'll be insuring against nutrient deficiency, you'll have less exposure to food allergy and you'll be much less likely to become bored.

Here's an amazing statistic: there are literally thousands of foods to select from but the average American consumes only about 12 to 15 foods. People tend to get stuck in eating routines, many of which are unhealthy, sometimes for years, sometimes even for life. Some of us learned our eating habits from our mothers and we've never had the joy of trying — and loving — something new. When we eat out, we tend to go to the same places and order the same things from the menu.

One survey found that people who were eating breakfast cereals, breads, rolls, crackers, muffins, spaghetti, cookies, cake and pretzels thought they were eating a variety of grains. In fact, they were eating various forms of wheat — and lots of it. It's well-known that wheat is one of the most allergenic foods we consume. When these people began replacing wheat with other grains like rice, millet, corn, oats and buckwheat, to name a few, they had dramatic positive results.

Food allergy is related not only to the amount consumed but also the frequency of consumption. If you eat the same foods every day, you're more likely to have allergic reactions. By the way, these reactions are not always dramatic, like hives or anaphylactic shock. Many times they're subtle, even undetectable, and they can have a profound effect on your energy and mood. This is an area where a nutritionist can really help you discover the good and bad of what you're eating.

Next time you're in the supermarket, an outdoor farmer's market or even a small ethnic grocery, look for something new. It might be a food or it might be a recipe. If it looks appealing, investigate its component parts. If it's healthy for you, buy it and try it. If you hate it, so be it. But ahhhh — if you love it, you'll have a new, healthy and delicious food! If variety is the spice of life, use it abundantly!

PRINCIPLE TWO: SIMPLICITY

There has been a great deal written about proper "food combining," including claims that mixing certain foods will cure everything from arthritis to obesity. And despite all the charts and rules to follow, there's no ultimate validation that food combining is the answer. That's not to say that food combining isn't healthful, it's only that the whole matter is much simpler than the "food combiners" would have you believe.

One rule of food combining is generally considered valid and that is that it's unwise to mix fruit with other foods. The reason is that fruit digests rapidly and it's a source of natural sugar. Combining it with other more complex foods keeps it in your system long after it has broken down, which may lead to fermentation and indigestion. So, eat your fruit on an empty stomach, such as in the morning and don't eat anything else for at least 20 to 30 minutes.

Here's a simple rule: Eat your food in the proper order, with the easiest to digest first and the most difficult to digest last. This stimulates and starts your system, "warms it up" and gets it ready for the main course.

Once you've begun a routine that suits you in taste and nutrition, don't be preoccupied with it. If it's weight loss you're seeking, don't run to the scale every morning with those high expectations that usually end in disappointment. Just let it be what it is. Hit the scale every month or so and I think you'll be pleasantly surprised. The main question is, "How do I feel?" If your energy levels are good and sustain you throughout the day, this is a good thing. If your energy flags in the late afternoon, you may need a simple protein boost around 3:00pm. That's all — simple.

Another way to simplify is to create meals which provide maximum nutrition from a minimum number of items. A "kitchen sink" salad, as I call it, with all kinds of tasty and healthy goodies in it can be as satisfying as a full course meal. You get the nutrition without the bulk, you get protein, fiber, vitamins, minerals, essential fats — and you do your digestive system a favor. Simple and delicious.

Talking about maximum nutrition with simplicity, there's another important rule to keep in mind. Whenever you can, with the exception of meats, fowl and fish, try to eat foods as close as possible to their natural state. If you over-boil your vegetables, for example, you'd be better off drinking the water you cooked them in, because that's where the nutrition is! Cook your veggies *al dente,* with a slight crispness to them, and they'll nourish you well. Of course, there's no better fiber than you get from raw carrots, celery, jicama, radishes and so on. Fruit should be eaten raw or steamed lightly. Simple and healthy.

PRINCIPLE THREE – MODERATION

The ancients Greeks called it "The Golden Mean". Simply put, it's "everything in moderation."

Moderate meals digest better than excessive ones. The fire of your digestive system, just like any other fire, quickly burns kindling and small branches but if you throw on a huge log, it smolders and soon goes out. In the same way, overeating leads to indigestion. The bloating and discomfort you feel are early-warning signs of greater trouble ahead, including premature aging. Indigestion increases the incidence and severity of food allergies. Slow digestion due to overeating causes fermentation and putrefaction, which, in turn produce a number of toxic by-products. Health professionals worldwide agree that moderation and proper chewing are the two most important components of healthy digestion. Digestion begins in the mouth. All you have to do is take smaller mouthfuls and chew them up completely before you swallow. Sounds simple — but when you're in a hurry or just plain famished, you tend to "wolf" your food. The fact is when you swallow half-chewed food, especially meat and other heavy things, you are putting an extra burden on your digestive system, and eventually you will pay a price.

It's no surprise that moderation is linked to longevity. One theory is that decreased caloric intake stimulates the immune system. The idea is that our evolution over the last 3.5 million years and our inconsistent food supply along the way, have affected our bodies in an interesting way. When we reduce our caloric intake, our bodies respond to what they perceive as impending starvation by turning to other resources of energy, such as stored fats, and by stimulating the immune system as a compensating strategy for survival.

There's much disagreement about how we can best take advantage of this evolutionary health boost. Some believe that fasting one or two days is necessary to activate this mechanism. Others believe that the same benefits can be obtained and maintained by controlled under-eating. I think it's all connected to our appetite.

Have you ever noticed when you're dining in an upscale restaurant that the dessert cart often appears before the main course dishes are cleared from the table? This is because the restauranteur knows that our appetites shut off about 12 minutes after we finish eating. If they bring the dessert 12-15 minutes later, we would turn them down saying, "No thanks, I'm stuffed!"

So moderate your food intake by controlling appetite. Take smaller portions, eat slowly, chew thoroughly and wait at least 10 minutes before you consider dessert. Also, your stomach is flexible and if you consistently eat large meals, your stomach will stretch to accommodate them. When you eat smaller portions and you don't stuff your stomach all day with snack foods between meals, your stomach will shrink and so will your appetite.

All the centenarians I have interviewed told me they eat moderate, simple, natural foods. Many of them said, "I eat when I'm hungry and when I'm no longer hungry, I stop." Good advice. For most people, eating has become a lifelong habit and they do it almost reflexively. Rarely do they give the actual way they eat any thought.

So here's an idea for you. For the next few meals, monitor your eating. Ask yourself: Did I eat more than I need? Did I "wolf" or chew? Did I need that dessert? At what point did my appetite subside? Am I helping my digestive system or putting undue strain on it? The answers will give you some clues about your own eating habits. I think you'll find the changes you make will be relatively easy.

PRINCIPLE FOUR – PURITY

The last principle of sensible, satisfying and no-nonsense eating is the purity of our food and water. The most nutritious foods, after all, will do us no good if they are not pure. Food should always be as fresh as possible and free from adulteration. Get genuine organically grown fruits and vegetables whenever you can. The benefit of protection from pesticide residue, preservatives and other additives is well worth the extra expense. If you buy non-organic, make sure you wash the produce thoroughly. There are several products on the market that are effective in removing most chemicals. Organic foods may not be more nutritious but they are certainly less harmful, especially in the long run.

You knew I was going to say this: avoid *all* processed foods! No less authority than the National Cancer Institute warns us of the long-term consequences of eating processed food. Here's another piece of advice you've heard before: read the labels on *everything* you buy to eat! You will often be shocked by what you find there. I once picked up a package of six smallish pastries because they looked delicious. Of course they were loaded with all kinds of bad stuff but what really got my attention was that each little pastry contained almost 1,000 calories!

Be cautious when buying meat and poultry. Some meat and poultry comes from animals that have been given so many chemicals, such as hormones, steroids and antibiotics, that eating them regularly can actually change your own hormone levels and blood chemistry. Mad Cow Disease is a serious danger. Likewise, seafood can contain mercury, lead and cadmium. In most cases, wild fish are safer than farm-grown and a great source of Omega 3. Otherwise, your best protection is asking questions. How fresh is this meat, poultry or fish? How were these animals fed? Where was this fish caught and when?

Most people are very aware by now that water purity is also of great importance. According to the Environmental Protection Agency, the municipal water supplies in many American cities are sub-standard. The cheapest and most effective way of assuring yourself that you're drinking and cooking with pure water is a good quality home purification system. Otherwise, keep well-filtered bottled water at hand at all times.

I think, as you take more care in selecting the things you put in your body, you will get a feeling of pride and satisfaction about taking better care of "number one." I think you'll feel better and look better too.

There are two important concepts that have been proven to be very effective in weight control and maintenance, as well as disease prevention.

Glycemic Index. This index charts how fast carbohydrates are converted into glucose and how rapidly the glucose causes the blood sugar to rise.

In my personal case, this was a happy answer for my struggle to lose my "spare tire." My belief had always been that vigorous exercise was enough to keep my body fat and blood sugar under control. The Glycemic Index taught me that the higher the glycemic load becomes, the greater the risk of developing obesity, silent inflammation and Diabetes.

After my yearly checkup, my blood sugar was

slightly elevated but high enough to scare me into changing my ways of eating.

Here's what I did. Coming from Scandinavia, my comfort foods — white pastas, white potatoes, white bread, croissants, white rice, — they were all high carb foods and they all had to go! My slogan became, "The less white I eat, the more fat I'll lose!"

Can you believe that sweet potatoes have less sugar than white potatoes? In the Glycemic Index chapter of "The New Sugar Busters®, The authors say, "a 6-ounce potato calculates to 22 teaspoons and a 10-ounce potato to 37 teaspoons of sugar!" Yikes! I love yams, so that was an easy one. Soft drinks and sweet juices were never favorites of mine, so they weren't a problem either. I substituted blueberries for watermelon, pears for ripe bananas and walnuts, sunflower seeds and pumpkin seeds for dates and raisins.

In the morning, I make myself fresh-squeezed lemon juice with a dash of cayenne pepper, which is a good blood cleanser. Also, once or twice per month, I do the following recipe in my juicer. I call it my "liver fix":

Juice of one organic lemon
2 celery sticks
¼ beet
1 cucumber
1 slice of ginger
¼ cup of water to dilute

It's important to drink it immediately while it's

foaming, so you get all the enzymes.

If you enjoy wine, remember it has lots of sugar in it. If you drink wine on an empty stomach, it absorbs incredibly fast and spikes your blood sugar. So, always drink wine with a meal. At the very least, if you can't eat a full meal, drink your wine with "a protein chaser", such as cheese, avocado, shrimp or chicken.

Silent Inflammation. Everybody knows that the inflammation and swelling from something like a sprained ankle cause pain. But silent inflammation is dangerous to your health and you aren't aware of it until its damage is done.

Several things cause silent inflammation in the cells, among them are stress, overweight and the body's production of too much insulin, cortisol and something called eicosanoids.

I lived at the beach for about nine months last year and I should have been a very happy camper — but I wasn't. My two beautiful daughters had just left home and I was suffering from Empty Nest Syndrome, I had unexplained aches and pains, I was moody and I had trouble sleeping. All of these things were either brand new for me or very unusual.

I started reading *The Anti Inflammation Zone, Reversing the Silent Epidemic That's Destroying Our Health"*, by Barry Sears, which a doctor friend of mine had given me. I decided I would take action immediately.

I started taking hour-long walks on the beach, combined with deep breathing techniques in the fresh ocean air. Next, I attacked my kitchen cupboards. I replaced sunflower and safflower oils with extra virgin olive oil. I ate grilled fresh fish, like salmon and halibut, two or three times per week with fresh vegetables and salads.

I have an unpleasant memory from my childhood of being forced to take cod liver oil, so the idea of taking fish oil was quite repugnant. I was relieved that, instead of an old tablespoon like my mother's, I could take it in capsule form. I started taking Omega-3 fatty acids with total EPA & DHA, as well as Salmon Oil and Omega-3 Flax Oil every day. I also took a teaspoon of Turmeric, a well-known natural anti-inflammatory, in a cup of low-fat yogurt as a mid-day snack.

In about three weeks to a month, I began to have more energy and vitality, I lost weight around my waist, I was sleeping better and my usual enjoyment of life returned.

* *

Recommended Reading & Websites

The Complete Idiot's Guide to Glycemic Index Weight Loss, Lucy Beale and Joan Clark, 2005, Penguin Books, available on Amazon.com

The New Sugar Busters!®, H. Leighton Steward, Morrison C. Bethea, M.D., Sam S. Andrews, M.D. and

Luis A. Balart, M.D., Ballantine Books, 2003, available on Amazon.com

The New Glucose Revolution: The Authoritative Guide To The Glycemic Index – The Dietary Solution For Lifelong Health, Marlowe & Co., 2007, available on Amazon.com

All Your Health Questions Answered, Maureen Kennedy Salaman, MKS, Inc., 1998, available on Amazon.com

Prescription For Nutritional Healing, 4th Edition: A Practical A-to-Z Reference to Drug-Free Remedies using Vitamins, Minerals, Herbs and Food Supplements, Phyllis A. Balch, Avery, 2006, available on Amazon.com

Foods That Heal, Dr. Bernard Jensen, Avery, 1988, 1993, available on Amazon.com

The Juicing Bible, Pat Crocker & Susan Eagles, Robert Rose, 2000, available on Amazon.com

Eating For Life: Your Guide To Great Health, Fat Loss and Great Energy!, Bill Phillips, High Pointe Media, 2003, available on Amazon.com

Sugar Shock!: How Sweets And Simple Carbs Can Derail Your Life — And How You Can Get Back On Track, Connie Bennett and Stephen Sinatra, Penguin Group, 2007, available on Amazon.com

Webmd.com

5 THE PERFECT WEIGHT AT ANY AGE

Suppose you could learn to eat in a way that would help you to achieve and maintain a perfect weight, avoid illness, postpone premature aging and even stretch your lifespan to 125 quality years. Would you make the change? What if it were delicious too? Would you change your ways?

This plan is a way of eating for the rest of your life, using common sense, some simple rules and a desire to look and feel your best. The really difficult part comes in the very beginning — the commitment.

First, be honest with yourself. This is not a fad diet. This is not a quick-fix. This is a permanent lifestyle change. The fun part is that you get to design it yourself according to your own tastes and nutritional needs. Remember, you've been eating one way for all your prior years and your eating habits are now subconscious. At any age, it takes at least 21 days to change a subconscious eating habit. Your body's going to be saying, "Hey! What are you trying to give me here?" The answer is healthful longevity. So be patient with yourself.

After your commitment is in place, make an effort to understand why you eat, when you eat and where you eat. Pay special attention to the times you overeat or eat in an unhealthy manner. We develop our individual relationships with food in childhood and they stay with us into adulthood. The food is often more varied and complex but the patterns are the same. If they're healthy — great. If they're not — we're in trouble.

Kids who were given sweets as a reward, tend to continue rewarding themselves in adulthood, whether they deserve it or not. Kids who got cookies and milk to bribe them into going to bed, tend to be late night sweet eaters. Some overeating is based in food punishment — "You're not leaving this table until you finish your lima beans!" Or food guilt — "There are millions of starving children in China who would love to eat those lima beans!" When my mother tried that one on me, I said, "Why don't we mail the lima beans to China?" The suggestion was not well received.

Food triggers the pleasure center of the brain, as do sex and certain drugs. If we use food as a substitute for something that's missing — such as love or self-esteem — this is where cravings and even addiction can start. Some people eat to be fat because they feel it is extra padding to protect them from all sorts of perceived hurts and disappointments. Eating, driven by psychological cravings, can please the brain and ultimately destroy the rest of the body. This is how a person can be grossly overweight and, at the same time, be seriously malnourished.

So, give some real thought to your own personal psychology of eating. Talk it over with your siblings and friends. Talk to a psychotherapist or a nutritionist with a specialty in eating disorders. You'll find yourself saying "ah, ha!" a lot and you'll get some important clues to help you design your own brand-new eating habit.

Now, you have a commitment to change your lifestyle permanently and knowledge of some of the psychology behind your life-long eating habits. It's time for the next step.

Chart your food intake for one full week. Keep a note pad handy at all times and write down every single thing you consume, including that handful of nuts, even that occasional stick of gum. A word of warning: don't censor yourself just because you're charting your food! Eat whatever you want, whenever you want and as much as you want. Make a note of how you're feeling when you order that second piece of pie or have that dish of ice cream before you go to bed. Do you feel guilty? Are you worried or anxious about something? Jot it down. All the cravings, all the "sins" — everything goes into your notes. Don't read your chart and notes until the end of the week. Remember, don't censor yourself.

At the end of the week, you will see what your eating is all about. You'll see the good, bad and the ugly. And you'll begin to get an idea of what you can change permanently for your good health and longevity.

I read an article by a nutritionist who worked with her clients on food replacement. She wrote about a grossly obese man who was suffering from a myriad of medical problems and who was desperate to lose weight. She took one look at his food chart and one item jumped off the page. This man was eating a pint of Haagen Dazs ice cream every night before he went to sleep! "So," she said, "let's start here!" She sent the man out to look for a fat-free frozen yogurt that really satisfied his taste buds. He found one and ate it every single night, just as he had done with the ice cream.

The weight just fell off him — almost 60 pounds! Why? He had reduced his caloric intake drastically at a very crucial time of the day. She reported that he became so excited with this success, that he found the motivation and desire to completely renovate his entire system of eating. It took almost two years for him to reach a healthy weight and, along the way, his medical problems receded and some disappeared entirely.

When you look over your eating chart, things will jump off the page at you too, hopefully not such dramatic ones. You'll find yourself saying, "Why in the world am I eating so much of that — I don't even like it that much!" Or, "No wonder I'm crashing at 11:00am — I'm loading my empty stomach with sugar first thing in the morning!"

Now, all you have to do is replace the offending foods or habits with healthy, nutritious and tasty ones. It's very likely that you won't feel deprived, you won't feel hungry. Instead, I think you'll find that you feel energized and excited about your new changes. And guess what? You're on your way to your perfect weight.

Here's a caution, though. Body image has gained an importance way beyond what it should be. So, at this stage of your renewal, be sure to set short-term and realistic goals for yourself. Don't get on the scale every day. Don't try to be a supermodel. Unrealistic expectations can lead to disappointments, which lead to discouragement, which leads to giving up. Let feeling and looking better be enough for now. Let your improving health excite and motivate you. Pat yourself on the back for every single step you take on your new path, no matter how small.

I guess you already know by now that changing your eating habits alone is not the complete solution. Of equal importance is regular exercise, because it stimulates muscle growth, faster metabolism and a positive mental attitude. Many people begin a diet and increase their exercise levels to speed up their progress. Then, when they achieve their goal, they make a classic mistake. They stop their diet and exercise regimen at the same time, which immediately sets them on the path right back to where they started.

We've talked about changing your eating habits permanently, so too must your regular exercise be for your lifetime. Just as you're your new food choices must be delicious and nutritious, so too must the exercise you choose for yourself be satisfying and enjoyable.

Some people enjoy exercising alone — working with moderate free weights, jogging long distances or rowing. They become ritualistic and feel deprived if they miss a day. It's easy for them to continue their routines for many years. Unfortunately, a great number of people exercise in spurts — they think of it as an unpleasant necessity and it's very easy for them to quit.

If exercise has not been a big part of your life, it's important to seek out a routine or sport which is fun for you. Take lessons, if available, and develop your skills. Develop a routine and stick to it — and, for Pete's sake have fun! You'll be much more likely to continue for a long time. My best advice is to find a group of like-minded people with a similar level of proficiency. Set a regular schedule and keep to it.

My husband and his friends have been playing men's doubles tennis every Tuesday and Thursday morning for over twenty years. If someone is sick or traveling, they have alternates who fill in for them so the games can continue. When a regular group of people is involved together in some sort of exercise, there is a special motivation to participate.

Now for those simple rules. These are mine — you can use them or make your own. The important thing is to make them positive, realistic and easy to follow. And believe in them. They are your guide to your perfect weight.

1. Avoid high salt intake foods. Use a healthy salt substitute if you need to, but go easy. If you aren't already doing so, read the nutrition stats on everything you buy. You'll be amazed what's in the food you eat.

2. Avoid high sugar intake. This doesn't just only mean candy bars and donuts. It means all the food that is prepared with sugar as an ingredient. If you need the taste of sugar, use the healthiest substitute you can find and use it sparingly. Sometimes the pancreas reacts to fake sugar as if it were real, which can cause low blood sugar. Again, read the labels.

3. Limit your alcohol intake to 1 – 2 drinks daily. Pay special attention to those drinks, like wine, that contain lots of sugar.

4. Replace your "trouble food" (you're in big trouble if you eat them!) with healthy, tasty, satisfying, nutritious things. Begin with the "trouble food" you really know you can live without and go from there.

5. Replace the "trouble food" in your fridge and kitchen cabinets with your favorite nutritious things. Remember, if you don't buy "trouble food", you're much less likely to eat it!

6. Spend more time with health-conscious people, meaning people who are more likely to eat a salad than a cheesecake. Or who actually play tennis instead of watching it on TV. There is such a thing as *positive* peer pressure, you know.

7. You've got to move to improve, so any time you can walk instead of drive, do it. Any time you can take the stairs instead of the elevator, do it.

8. If you need a reward for good behavior, instead of food, reward yourself with a facial or a massage or any health-promoting thing you enjoy. That way, your reward is a reward in itself.

9. Stay off the scale. Your clothes, especially your belt, will tell you you're making progress.

10. As you approach your perfect weight, when the time is right, buy some clothes in a smaller size that fit you well and tailor or toss out some of your "fat clothes"! Let your clothes be your scale. They'll let you know when you're thinning or spreading a little. Never, I repeat NEVER buy a larger size. It's so much easier to lose 10 pounds than 50!

Monitoring blood sugar is crucial for people with diabetes. The Glycemic Index was developed to help them understand how certain foods are absorbed into their bloodstream as glucose. Glucose that isn't burned by the body through daily activity is stored in the body as fat. Some foods cause a rapid rise in blood sugar, others cause a moderate or slow rise in blood sugar. Nowadays, dieticians, nutritionists and weight loss experts are using the Glycemic Index to help reduce cravings, unnatural hunger and to control glucose levels.

Likewise, you can develop an understanding of how your body absorbs the foods you eat with a special focus on blood sugar. Also, consider adding cinnamon in powder or pill form to your food intake, because it is effective in lowering blood sugar levels.

If you have a problem believing you can be successful, work on it. As you make progress, no matter how small, allow yourself more and more to believe in your ultimate success. Work on your motivation too. Keep a photo of yourself at your perfect weight in a frame by your bed or your fridge. Find a "buddy" to join you on your road to your perfect weight. Study together, exercise together, discuss ideas, motivate, encourage and compliment each other.

Every night, just before you fall asleep, you can re-program your internal "computer" by saying to yourself, "It's easy and effortless for me to achieve and maintain my perfect weight." This may sound a little silly to you, but believe me, it works.

* *

Recommended Reading & Websites

YOU, The Owner's Manual: An Insider's Guide to the Body That Will Make You Healthier and Younger, Michael F. Roizen and Mehmet Oz, 2005, available on Amazon.com

The Anti-Inflammation Zone: Reversing the Silent Epidemic That's Destroying Our Health, Barry Sears, Regan, 2006, available on Amazon.com

Astaxanthin, Natural Astaxanthin: King of the Carotenoids, Bob Capelli, Cyanotech Corporation, 2007

The Herbal Drugstore, Linda B. White and Steven Foster, Rodale, 2003 available on Amazon.com

Eating Well For Optimum Health, Andrew Weil, Quill 2001

Seven Pillars Of Health, Don Colbert and Mary Colbert, Siloam, 2007, available on Amazon.com

Eating For Life: Your Guide To Great Health, Fat Loss and Great Energy!, Bill Phillips, High Pointe Media, 2003, available on Amazon.com

The Weight Loss Cure They Don't Want You To Know About, Kevin Trudeau, Alliance, 2007

6 MOVEMENT MAKES IMPROVEMENT

For millions of years mankind has worked hard to survive. The hunt for food consumed almost every waking moment. We spent most of our time outdoors, breathing fresh air and dodging predators. Our normal lifespan was very short.

Today, we have some sort of food on every corner. We have no predators to fear, that is, the kind that wish to eat us. We live and work in climate–controlled buildings. It's ironic, but it seems our incredible and ever-advancing technology is interfering with our biology. Our lifespan is much longer and the most dangerous predator we face is disease.

Children love to play. From the moment they learn to walk, most kids are in constant motion. They run, jump, climb trees. Sadly, some spend too much time in front of the TV, idly snacking on really bad food. These children are often overweight, out of shape and unmotivated. Why? They stopped moving.

Likewise our adult lifestyle, with all its stress and anxiety, tends to slow us down. Many jobs require us to sit for hours chained to a computer or standing at a checkout counter or an assembly line repeating the same motions over and over. We go home tired, sit in front of the TV and eat really bad food.

The difference is that when adults, especially people over 50, live a sedentary lifestyle, it causes many to fall prey to obesity, arthritis, arteriosclerosis, heart disease, osteoporosis, diabetes, hypertension, constipation and depression. Why? Because the circulation of blood, lymph and cerebrospinal fluid depends on movement.

We all know the heart pumps blood, but good circulation requires more than a heartbeat. It needs a clean and efficient circulatory system. Good circulation means clean and healthy lungs to ensure that life-giving oxygen reaches all our cells.

Then there's the lymph system. Think of it as the sewer system of the body, which filters and disposes of many toxic elements, like the dead white blood cells which have fought and died to maintain our immunity to Nature's invaders and life's poisons. There's more lymphatic fluid in our bodies than there is blood. It is the heart of our immune system and it is critical to our survival. But there's a problem: no pump. Lymph relies on movement to circulate.

It's the same with the cerebrospinal fluid found in our spinal cord. It nourishes the central nerve channels of our body and it bathes and maintains the spongy discs between our vertebrae. It, too, is a critical part of our physiology and it, too, requires movement to flow. No wonder the less we move, the stiffer we get.

So, if you want to get better and feel younger, GET MOVING!

One out of every seven people in the U.S. suffers from some form of painful arthritis. A great deal of this pain could be alleviated or completely prevented by simple full-range-of-motion exercises. My simple program is designed to dramatically increase circulation of blood, lymph and cerebrospinal fluid.

Each twist, stretch, bend or simple posture uses the force of gravity to increase the flow of all these vital fluids.

Our bodies are constantly changing. We're growing older it's true. But the good news is our regenerative processes are continually at work, re-building every cell during our entire life. A balanced fitness program that includes nutritional, mental, emotional and spiritual factors boosts and supports those processes and anti-aging begins.

Design your exercise program to be both a workout and a "work-in." A safe and sane aerobic exercise workout strengthens and builds muscle and improves circulation. Your "work-in" should consist of slow and gentle movements combined with deep breathing, guided imagery, aroma therapy or anything which promotes deep relaxation within you. Your "work-in" helps you release deep-seated emotional stress, promotes a feeling of well-being and connects your body and mind in a special way.

"Where do I begin?" you ask. "Am I too old? Too fat? Too out of shape?" It's never too late to begin and everyone — I repeat — everyone can move and improve!

Just as with a weight loss program, your exercise program should begin with an emphasis on safety and realistic expectations. If you never walk at all, a 20 minute walk at a reasonable pace will bring you almost immediate results. Don't overdo it. Just do it, enjoy it and go from there. If you already do regular exercise, you know where you need the extra emphasis. It might be endurance or flexibility. Add these elements to your program slowly and gently. When you begin to feel your body and mind developing together, it is truly an amazing experience.

I have just a few cautions for you.

Please check with your doctor. I recommend a physical to check for conditions like hypertension, high cholesterol and others, so you can choose your program accordingly and feel safe and confident.

During exercise, if you ever feel any pain, stop what you're doing and rest. If you feel discomfort, just slow down and take it easy. Most of the time these things are temporary and it's always better to err on the conservative side.

Make sure you exercise in a safe and supportive place. If home is too hectic or distracting, find a spa or a group of like-minded people who exercise in a non-competitive environment.

When you design your program, keep in mind that exercise works simultaneously on three levels:

1. The outer physical, by increasing your strength, flexibility, muscle tone and balance.

2. The inner physical, by enhancing your circulation and toning and supporting all your organs and glands.

3. The mental, emotional and spiritual, by giving you relaxation, ease and harmony.

I'll give you a few suggestions for exercise in the next chapter but we can only scratch the surface. Check out the possibilities, try a few if you like, and then choose things you really like to do. Do them regularly, alone or with a buddy, enjoy what you do and focus on the process – not the results.

It's a funny thing but it's usually family and friends who first notice the change in you. You'll hear somebody say, "Did you lose weight?" or "You look great — what are you doing?" What's better than that?

* *

Recommended Reading & Websites

Fit For Life, Harvey and Marilyn Diamond, Warner, 1985, available on Amazon.com

Getting Back In Shape, 3rd Edition: 32 Workout Programs For Lifelong Fitness, Anderson, Pearl, Burke, Galloway, Shelter, 2007, available on Amazon.com

Stretching: 20th Anniversary, Bob Anderson, Shelter 2000

Yoga Minibook For Weight Loss, Elaine Gavalas, Fireside/Simon & Schuster, 2003, available on Amazon.com

7 SLIMMING DOWN, FIRMING UP

There are so many forms of exercise in our world today, it's a bit overwhelming. Infomercials trumpet the latest fad or exercise contraption. Are these things self-improvement or self abuse? If you use this new equipment without supervision will you hurt yourself?

I believe the key to slimming down and firming up is choosing an exercise that emphasizes muscle toning with little danger of injury. Whenever possible, learn techniques from qualified instructors to help ensure your safety. I think of muscle toning as working on that inner "hardbody" that's waiting to be revealed as your nutrition program continues. When you focus on toning exercise, you will notice results in your shape long before you reach your weight loss goal.

Here are a few safe and effective exercises to consider:

WALKING: At least 15 minutes at a brisk pace with lots of arm movement is a relatively gentle and effective way to drop pounds and increase muscle tone. If you wish, and you are in pretty good aerobic condition, you can add light hand and ankle weights to increase your calorie consumption. Solo walkers love to listen to upbeat music as they go. I recommend putting together a group of friends and setting a regular schedule. Conversation and laughter makes the time fly by. Also, the group can nag you when you don't feel like hauling yourself out of bed or off the couch! Drink water before, during and after your walks.

HIKING: Begin with relatively flat terrain and only a few hills to climb. Hiking puts more stress on your knees and ankles, so be careful. If you're hiking with others, please don't feel embarrassed if you need to stop and rest. It shouldn't be a competition, just a great day in Nature's playground. Drink water before, during and after your hikes.

SWIMMING: If you like to swim, this is one of the most efficient over-all exercises. Begin by holding onto the side of the pool and kicking your legs vigorously until you become slightly winded. Then do several laps using your favorite stroke. I like the Breast Stroke with a frog kick and the good old Australian Crawl. Even though you're in water, drink water before and after your swim. (Yes, you CAN dehydrate in a swimming pool!)

PILATES: Pilates was developed by fitness expert Joseph Pilates in the 1940's and only hit the mainstream a few years ago. It can be done on the floor or with equipment especially designed for it. It is an excellent toning exercise but it should always be done under the watchful eye of a highly competent instructor. Drink water before, during and after your workout.

CORE TRAINING: This very popular program focuses work on the center of the body, front, back and sides. If your waistline hasn't made an appearance for a long while, Core Training is a good way to rediscover it. But, for heaven's sake, be sensible about these more intense workouts. Begin gently, progress slowly and carefully and don't overdo it. If you're laid up for a few weeks with an injury, it's very discouraging. A good instructor will not use insults and humiliation to motivate you. If they do, run right out of there and find a better teacher! And, yes, drink water before, during and after your Core Training session.

INTEGRAL YOGA: This ancient system of postures is designed to improve and maintain one's mental, physical and spiritual well-being. Yoga is not Hindu Mysticism. It's a philosophy and a way of life. I learned Hatha Yoga with Sri Swami Satchidananda at his Integral Yoga Institute in Los Angeles. I have taught Yoga for more than 25 years to literally thousands of students. I train teachers to pass along the knowledge given to me by my teacher. My youngest student was 3 and my oldest is 106. I teach people with all sorts of health challenges, like Parkinson's, MS, Lupus and Arthritis.

I hope you'll believe me when I say that everyone — young or old, healthy or health-challenged, big or small, spry or lame — they all improved their health and well-being with a simple, beginner to intermediate Yoga practice. For those that may not have had the chance to try Yoga, I'd like to offer a brief overview of this wonderful feast for body and soul.

First, find a class appropriate for your age and physical condition. Make sure your teacher is certified by a qualified teacher or school. My teacher, Swami Satchidananda, helped found the Yoga Alliance which sets minimum standards for teachers and registers them. If you see the letters RYT (Registered Yoga Teacher) after your teacher's name, you can feel secure that you are in good hands.

Your classes will focus on proper balance, spinal alignment and Pranayama, the science of breath, without which Yoga would be just a stretch class. I recommend you take at least two classes per week so you can achieve results quicker and progress faster. Your classes will feature twists, forward and backward bending, balancing and plenty of deep breathing. Yoga does more than strengthen and tone your muscles. It guides you to a central place in your spiritual being and it helps you develop the inner strength you need to accomplish all sorts of things. Some of my students have stopped smoking, others have overcome negative personality traits, such as road rage. One woman found the strength to end her long, unhappy marriage and find a new, joyful and rewarding life!

Practically all of my students over the years have had one challenge in common: stress. I'm sure they would agree with me that Yoga is the single greatest natural defense against stress and anxiety there is, hands down. And once again, please take a bottle of water to Yoga class.

****

Recommended Reading & Websites

Walking: The Ultimate Exercise For Optimum Health, Andrew Weil and Mark Fenton, 2006, available on Amazon.com

Getting Back In Shape, 3rd Edition: 32 Workout

Programs For Lifelong Fitness, Anderson, Pearl, Burke, Galloway, Shelter, 2007, available on Amazon.com

Core Performance Essentials: The Revolutionary Nutrition and Exercise Plan Adapted For Everyday Use, Mark Verstegen, Pete Williams, Rodale, 2006, available on Amazon.com

Pilates, Rael Isacowitz, Human Kinetics, 2006, available on Amazon.com

The Fit Swimmer: 120 Workouts and Training Tips, Marianne Brems, 1984, available on Amazon.com

8 STRESS REDUCTION EQUALS LIFE EXTENSION

There are many definitions of stress. I like this one: "Stress is any demand made upon your nervous system." Any demand. This means stress can be positive and negative. Running to catch a train that's taking you to your cruise ship for a two week holiday on the Caribbean Sea is stressful. Running to catch the last train that will get you to work on time, ah … that's a very different kind of stress.

In our modern society we are forced to hurry, rush, speed and run 'til we pant. A good deal of the time we're hurrying to do things we neither believe in nor enjoy. We worry, struggle, compete, defend, labor, fight and endure all sorts of hardships and disappointments. We still have our cavemen ancestors' "fight or flight" mechanism but in our modern world, flight is rarely a viable option. Unless we have a way of releasing ourselves daily from stress's death grip, it can literally kill us.

Remember the movie "NETWORK"? The people run to their windows, stick their heads out and yell, "I'm mad as Hell and I'm not going to take it anymore!" Why can't we do that?

The reasons are many.

Societal brainwashing, traditional family influences, fear, survival, greed, ignorance, the need for approval, the need to please others, or just a pervasive feeling of being powerless — they all make it easier for us to succumb to so many negative demands on our bodies and minds. Stress saps energy, lowers our immune systems, alters our moods and deprives us of sleep. Unless we find ways to release stress, and its constant companions, anxiety, tension and depression, it will destroy us from within.

But do we even have a chance? A choice in the matter? You bet. The choice is always ours. We can make changes, small and large, in our lifestyles and attitudes that move us toward more productive, happy, healthy and fulfilling lives. Did you notice I didn't say "stress-free?" Sadly, our lives will never be stress-free. But we can CONQUER stress.

Fighting stress is stressful. Understanding stress and our own relationship to it is the key. Creating and developing our own system of successfully managing and releasing stress is very empowering.

So let's talk a little about the effects of negative stress and tension on your body, mind and spirit.

Chronic stress without relief changes your body chemistry. Your glands don't know how to think, they just react. Under stress, your pituitary gland, also known as The Master Gland, secretes adreno-cortitropic hormones which may result in lowering your sex drive. The adrenal glands secrete glucocorticoids which can lead to higher blood sugar levels. The thyroid gland secretes thyroxine which speeds up your metabolism.

Most people are so "uptight" that they are not even aware of their stress level. A new Yoga student of mine was complaining of insomnia and wanted to know if deep relaxation would help her sleep. I asked her if she was feeling a lot of stress and tension during the day. Her answer has always stuck in my mind. She said, "No more than normal." No more than normal? That suggests it's somehow normal to go through your day feeling stressed. It's not.

Mass media advertising seems to work very hard to convince us that stress-caused headaches, indigestion, muscle soreness and heartburn are normal. Millions of people come home from work after a busy day, slump into a favorite chair and say, "I'm exhausted!" Are they exhausted from physical labor? Some are, of course. The fact is that many, many people spend their entire workday seated in a chair, chained to a computer. I believe the principal causes of their "exhaustion" are inactivity and tension. Just the simple act of maintaining your head, neck and shoulders in the same position for extended periods saps a lot of energy. Lack of movement throughout the day causes shallow breathing, slows lymph flow, slows circulation in the extremities, and leads to a feeling of lethargy.

But there's more bad news. When you're tense, your muscles tighten and your energy pathways become blocked. You tend to retain toxins and waste, which leads to constipation. Under relentless tension, your body has difficulty assimilating cholesterol which leads to arterial blockage. The increased production of adrenaline and cortisol can lead to hypertension and heart damage.

There are many very powerful "stressors" in our world, such as career building, college for the kids, maintaining relationships with bosses, co-workers, family and friends, social activities. And for Baby

Boomers, illness, death of a spouse, children leaving the home (Empty Nest Syndrome), retirement and parenting elderly parents are all enormously stressful. It's all very real, dangerous and harmful to our health.

Now for some good news. Positive stress is the result of our creativity, our dreams and goals. It's the healthy response to life's challenges that motivates us to advance. It arises from the excitement we feel as we use and develop our talents and skills. Without the stimulus of our positive stress, we couldn't get very much done. Positive stress is our friend and we should welcome and nurture it. Likewise, negative stress is the enemy, hell-bent on killing us and we should learn to manage it.

How do we tell the difference? Introspection. When you're feeling stressed, develop the habit of stopping, feeling and thinking about what's going on. If you're nervous about the speech you have to give but excited about giving it — positive stress. If you're nervous about the speech and fearful about giving it because you know you're unprepared — negative stress. Work hard on your preparation and turn your negative stress to positive.

As we grow up, life brings us more and more stress. Spelling tests, math tests, mean kids on the playground. Junior High and High School bring more academic stress, raging hormones and the eternal mystery of dating and figuring out the other sex. Then it's college or university and more stress — not just good grades, term papers, theses and more dating — now it's preparing for career, marriage, kids and the rest of your life. Whew!

Think about it for a moment — with the possible exception of naptime in kindergarten, our education fails to give us even a hint of how to manage our stress. Most of us learn about stress and how to react to it from observing others. I guess you know this is not always a good thing. Suddenly, we're adults. We're in therapy and popping anti-depressants, sleeping pills and antacids, just trying to calm down.

My best advice is, if you haven't already done so, put yourself first. Your physical and spiritual health, your sense of well-being, your peace of mind must be nurtured and protected. When you're right with yourself and the world, you're the best you can be for everything you do. This is not selfishness, this is self-defense.

The first step is to get to the heart of what's causing your negative stress. Some people know exactly what's "eating" them. Others need professional guidance to sort it all out. Either way, once you identify the source, you're half way to managing or even eliminating your stress.

Some problems are like immovable objects. No matter how hard you shove, they just won't budge. Sometimes it's a job, sometimes a relationship, sometimes it's even a city — but in your heart you know they are the principal source of your stress and they are taking you nowhere. The easy part is finding a new job, a new mate or a new city. The hard part is making the decision to take action in defense of your happiness and peace of mind. Once the decision is made in your heart and mind and you take the first step toward positive change, it's like a heavy load is lifted off your shoulders. This is major stress relief.

But what about that daily assault by all those minor stressors like car trouble, dropped cell phone calls, late for work and low on gas, and bumper-to-bumper traffic? The so-called "normal, everybody's-got it-stress"? When it accumulates, without relief, it will wear you out and sap every bit of your positive energy.

Keep in mind that relaxation and stress can't exist together inside you at the same time. Here are a few things you can do to bring more deep relaxation into your life.

1. Be more aware of how you feel. Work on taking what we might call your "emotional temperature." Are you reasonably calm or are red lights flashing and sirens blaring?

2. Carve out quality time for yourself. An hour per day is best but even 20 good, quiet minutes will work. Just be sure they are yours and yours alone. After all, there are 24 hours in each day — why can't you have just one for yourself?

3. Take a nap. This means take off your shoes, get horizontal, close your eyes, deep breathe and relax. Don't take off more than your shoes and don't get under the covers. Your body may think you're going to sleep for the night and you'll sleep too deeply.

4. Keep a journal of your thoughts and stresses. It's well known that externalizing these kinds of thoughts can remove a great deal of their negative impact on your subconscious mind.

5. Take a deep muscle massage at least once per week. Your neck, shoulders and lower back hold a

large percentage of your tension.

6. Add some kind of energetic fun to your life, fun being the key word. Dancing, swimming, tennis, golf, yoga — anything which can help you burn off your tension and nervous energy.

7. Take brief, periodic "stress breaks" during the day. I'd like to offer you several of these amazing stress management techniques, with a special focus on the areas where stress most often accumulates. If they seem simple, it's only because they are!

EYES: Our eyes are the most neglected of our five senses, even though some 60% of our nervous tension passes through them. They are constantly focusing, adapting to light changes and moving rapidly as we perceive the outside world. Each eye has six muscles to control all the movements and an optic nerve to send signals to the brain. I always tell my patients and students, "Don't take your eyesight for granted." We stretch, exercise and relax all our other muscles but we don't have a clue what to do to our poor, over-worked eyes. Until now, that is! Do this simple routine as needed throughout the day and feel the difference when you get home:

1. Keep your spine straight and your head still as you look straight ahead. Now, slowly roll your eyes upward and downward. Repeat 5 times. Close your eyes for a few seconds, then open and blink rapidly a few times.

2. Now, keep your head still and look all the way to the right and all the way to the left. Repeat 5 times. Again, close your eyes for a few seconds, then open

and blink a few times.

3. Look up toward the ceiling and roll your eyes slowly to the right, or clockwise, as though you're counting all the numbers on the clock 1 to 12. When you reach 12 o'clock, roll your eyes slowly counter-clockwise all the way around. Repeat 3 times each way. Close your eyes and rest for a few moments. Now, with your eyes closed, rub your palms together firmly and briskly for awhile. When the friction begins to create heat in your palms, gently cup them over your eyes, inhale and exhale deeply as you absorb the soothing energy. Now, blink your eyes a few times and feel how the tension has left them.

NECK: Over 65 million people suffer from a "pain in the neck", literally. There just is no way to get through the day without aggravating our neck and shoulder muscles. Think of your head as a 14 pound bowling ball, supported by your neck and shoulder muscles. When your head is held straight and balanced, no problem. The minute you bend forward, your neck and shoulder muscles have to hold up this 14 pound weight. Problem! By practicing this easy routine often, you can banish neck tension and pain once and for all:

1. Inhale deeply and with your eyes open, gently drop your head backward. Don't strain. Hold for a few seconds. As you exhale deeply, drop your head gently forward. Repeat several times.

2. Inhale deeply and turn your head to the right as far as you can comfortably and hold for a few seconds. Exhale deeply as you turn your head back to center. Now do the same movement and breathing to

your left and back to center. Repeat several times on both sides.

3. Inhale and look upward. As you exhale, roll your head gently clockwise, ending your exhale as you reach "12 o'clock". Now inhale and roll your head back slowly counter-clockwise. Repeat several times on both sides.

SHOULDERS: I call the shoulders "the shock absorbers for tension". When you're happy and energetic, you hold your shoulders straight. When you're tired, your shoulders slump forward and feel stiff and sore. Chronic tension in the shoulders is a causal factor in many headaches and, in certain men, it can be a contributing factor in strokes. Serious business. Take a couple of minutes a few times per day to do this simple routine:

1. Stand or sit with your arms at your sides. Make a fist with your right hand, Inhale and bring your right shoulder up toward your right ear and hold firmly for a few seconds. Exhale and release. Make a fist with your left hand and inhale as you bring your left shoulder up toward your left ear and hold firmly for a few seconds. Exhale and release. Repeat on both sides 3 times.

2. Make fists with both hands and raise both shoulders up toward your ears. Hold firmly for a few seconds, exhale and release. Repeat 3 times.

3. Raise both arms out to the side to shoulder level with your palms up. Bend your elbows and touch your fingertips to your shoulders. Now, bring your elbows forward until they touch. Inhale deeply

as you raise your elbows slowly, upward and, then exhale as they lower behind you and return to the front. Feel the stretch. Repeat 5 times.

Now, roll your elbows downward and backward. Inhale as they come upward and return to the front. Exhale as they roll again downward and backward and inhale as they raise and return to the front. Repeat 5 times.

BACK: Your back is the support system for your entire body and you are exactly as healthy as your spine is. If you're a Babyboomer, you are most likely in the 80% of the American population that has experienced severe back pain. You'd be amazed how many people have never learned how to protect their backs. Here are a few tips for you, just in case. Think before you lift something heavy and give yourself a chance to change your mind. Bend your knees and lift with your legs, even if it's something as light as the morning paper. When getting into your car, put your backside in first — it's easier on your back. Ease into a chair, don't drop — less lower back compression. And last but not least, strong abdominals will help keep your lower spine in alignment — so work on those abs!

Stress and tension are often causes of chronic back pain. If you spend much of your day seated, I'll bet your back gets stiff and achy. All pain is a warning that something is wrong. Some reactions to pain stimuli are reflexive. When we burn ourselves on a hot stove, we instantly move away. We tend to ignore backaches and low back stiffness in that same "everybody's-got-'em" way. Let me say this to you in no uncertain terms, "When your body speaks to you, listen and take quick action to correct the problem." I'm going to give you a few Yoga-based routines that will help strengthen and relax your back muscles and keep your spine in good alignment.

1. Lie flat on the floor or on your bed, making sure you're comfortable and your back is straight. Inhale and raise your bent right knee toward your chest. Place your hands around your knee and pull it toward you as far as you can comfortably. Don't strain. Hold for a few seconds. Exhale and lower your leg back down. Repeat with your left knee. Now repeat 2 more times with each leg.

2. Now inhale and raise both legs, with your knees bent, toward your chest. Put both hands around your knees and pull them toward your chest as far as you can comfortably. Don't strain. Hold for a few seconds. Exhale and lower your legs back down. Repeat 2 more times.

3. Lie on your back with your knees bent, soles of your feet on the floor and your arms at your sides. Inhale and press down on your feet, raising your hips up as high as you can comfortably. Place your palms on your lower back to help support your spine. Squeeze your buttocks tightly and hold a few seconds. Now, remove your palms and exhale as you slowly lower your back down to the floor. Repeat 2 more times and remember — don't strain.

4. Lie down on your stomach, face down. Bring your heels together to align your spine. Place your forehead on the floor. Place your palms on the floor, fingertips even with your shoulders. Inhale and bring your head up. Allow your lower back muscles to take

most of the effort. Hold a few seconds. Exhale and lower slowly back to the floor, vertebra by vertebra. If there is any pain at all, please stop immediately.

Yoga is a wonderful exercise because it is done slowly with deep breathing, and because it emphasizes posture, balance and alignment. If you haven't done so already, I hope you'll begin a series of classes with an experienced teacher.

Pay attention to your posture as often as you can during the day. Are you standing straight? Are you walking with your head up and shoulders back? If you are, I guarantee you you'll be looking and feeling younger and your spine will be happy.

****

Recommended Reading & Websites

How To Stop Worrying and Start Living, Dale Carnegie, Pocket Books/Simon & Schuster, 1984, 2007, available on Amazon.com

The Relaxation and Stress Reduction Workbook, Martha Davis, Matthew McKay, New Harbinger, 2000, available on Amazon.com

Adrenal Fatigue: The 21st-Century Stress Syndrome, James L. Wilson and Jonathan V. Wright, 2000, available on Amazon.com

Coping With Terrorism: Dreams Interrupted, Carole Lieberman, M.D., European-Atlantic Publications,

2006, www.copingwithterrorism.com

Ulla Anneli's The Break™, relieve stress and repetitive stress injuries with brief, easy-to-follow video exercise routines on your PC at home or work, **www.TakeTheBreak.com**

9 STRESS BREAKS AND ENERGY BOOSTERS

"I HAVE NO TIME TO DO EXERCISES!" is the most common complaint I hear from people. Well, the fact of the matter is that when you're busy, that's the time you really need to take a few minutes to relax, unwind and re-charge your batteries. What you do for yourself to beat stress every day is what counts most in the long run. You *can* find the time, you know. Why not make one of your coffee breaks a stress break?

Don't wait for the weekend or your annual vacation to relax. Do it right now. A few breaks spread throughout your day will help prevent stress build-up and mental fatigue. Your muscles will have a chance to clear themselves of the waste that causes physical fatigue. And your mind will benefit from the positive visualization you bring to your routines.

First the short breaks. Here are a few tried-and-true routines for you to try:

1. **IMMUNE SYSTEM BOOST**. Your Thymus gland is located just under your breast bone and when it is stimulated, it can literally awaken your sleepy immune system and improve its function, by increasing production of white blood cells. Some call the thymus the "fountain of youth."

Make a fist with your right hand and firmly tap your breast bone for about 30 seconds. At the same time, if you can, make a humming sound with a good strong voice. In Yoga practice we use the sound of "OM" (it rhymes with "home"). You can actually feel your breast bone vibrating with the taps and the sound.

2. **THE 5-MINUTE ENERGIZER**. Need a quick pick-me-up? Forget coffee. Forget the candy bar. Try this:

One Minute: Calming Breath. (Chapter 2, p. 20)

One Minute: Inhale and tense up your fists, arms and chest muscles and hold for a few seconds. Exhale and relax, releasing your tension.

One Minute: Roll your shoulders forward a few times, then backward a few times. Breathe deeply throughout. Feel the tension leaving your shoulders.

One Minute: With your eyes open, roll your head around slowly to the left three times. Then roll your head around slowly to the right. Breathe deeply throughout. Feel the tension leave your neck.

One Minute: Energy Breath. (Chapter 2, pp. 17, 18)

Now take a moment to become aware of the results. I think you'll be pleasantly surprised.

3. **FORWARD BEND**: This is great when you only have one or two minutes. Inhale and raise your hands high over your head. Look up at your fingers. Now, with your knees bent to protect your lower back, exhale and bend forward slowly, pointing your fingers toward your toes. Go as far as you can comfortably. Then, inhale and slowly straighten your back vertebra by vertebra, returning to your original

position. Exhale and relax. Repeat three times and don't strain.

****

DEEP RELAXATION: This is the most effective and powerful technique for removing stress, tension and anxiety from your body, mind and spirit. For this you will need a private, quiet and comfortable place, indoors or out, where you will not be disturbed for at least 20 minutes. That means no phones. I know this is tricky for many people but it is well worth the effort.

The following movements of body and breath are all one deep relaxation routine. I recommend that you record the routine in your own voice so you can follow it completely and in sequence without referring to the text.

It's best to lie on a carpet rather than a bed or a sofa. Loosen any constricting clothing, unbuckle your belt and remove your watch.

Lie on your back with your feet about 18 inches apart and your arms at your sides a few inches from your body, palms up. With your eyes closed, begin to breathe slowly and deeply. The breath should be unforced, comfortable and rhythmic. When you're ready, begin with the following movements and finish with the body visualization exercise:

LEG RAISES: Take a few moments to observe your breathing, then focus your attention on your right foot and leg. As you inhale, raise your right leg just three inches off the floor and tighten your leg muscles as much as you can comfortably. Hold for a few seconds, then release your breath completely and drop your leg abruptly back to the floor. Now roll your right foot gently from side to side and let it rest. Now repeat with your left leg and foot, paying special attention to your breathing.

ARM RAISES: Bring your attention to your right arm and hand. Stretch your fingers wide open and then curl them into a fist. As you inhale, raise your right arm up about three inches and clench your fist as tight as you can. Hold for a few seconds, then exhale and release completely, letting your arm drop back to the floor. Now roll your hand gently back and forth and let it rest. Now repeat with your left arm and hand.

Now feel that your legs and arms are getting heavier and heavier. Pretend they are so heavy you can't lift them off the floor. They are very relaxed.

BUTTOCK SQUEEZE: Now bring your attention to your buttocks. Inhale and tighten the muscles and feel your body lifting slightly. Hold for a few seconds, then exhale and release.

ROUND BELLY: Concentrate on your abdomen. Inhale very deeply and push your abdomen outward, like a balloon. Hold, then release your abdomen with a complete exhalation through your mouth.

CHEST EXPANSION: Inhale as deeply as you can, filling your chest completely, feeling your ribcage expand. Hold, then exhale deeply through your mouth.

SHOULDER SQUEEZE: Next, inhale and press your shoulders back, bringing your shoulder blades closer together. Hold a few moments, then exhale and relax. Now inhale and move your shoulders upward, widening the space between your shoulder blades. Hold a few moments, then exhale and relax.

FACE FLEX: Roll your head gently from side to side a few times. Center your head and bring your attention to the muscles of your face. "Scrunch" up all your face muscles — forehead, eyes and jaw. Hold for a few seconds, then release. Now, with your eyes closed, arch your eyebrows up as high as you can, open your mouth as wide as you can and stick out your tongue as far as it will go. Hold a few moments, then release. Feel the rush of fresh circulation to your face.

Now take a few moments to feel how your muscles have relaxed and your stress and tension are melting away.

BODY VISUALIZATION: This is done by keeping your body completely still and using only the healing power of your mind. (If you've never done this before, don't worry — this power has always been there, even if you've never used it consciously!).

Begin by visualizing a wave of relaxing energy flowing into your toes, rolling over the bottoms and tops of your feet up to your ankles, shin and calves. Feel the wave of soothing energy massaging your knees, front and back, and your thighs. Remain completely relaxed as you bring your attention to your fingers, hands and arms.

Feel the relaxing energy flowing into your fingers, rolling over your palms and the backs of your hands, coming up your wrists to your forearms, elbows and upper arms. Take a moment to feel the relaxation.

Now, bring this same wave of relaxation into your pelvic area, relaxing your groin muscles and buttocks. Feel it flowing up into your abdomen, lower back, stomach and the middle of your back. Let it flow into your chest, relaxing the lungs and heart. Feel this soothing energy flowing up your back to your shoulders and up the back of your neck, releasing tension as it moves.

Now the healing energy enters your head, first to your throat and mouth, relaxing your jaws and lips. If your tongue is pressed against the roof of your mouth, allow it to relax. Focus your attention on your face. Relax your cheeks eyes, eyelids, the area behind your eyes, your temples and then up to your forehead and the top of your head.

At this point you are entering into a profound and restful awareness. Laboratory instruments measuring the subtle electrical energy of the nervous system have verified that an individual in this state may achieve a greater degree of relaxation than that provided by a deep sleep.

Turn your attention to your breath. Don't try to breathe in any specific way. Just witness your breath as it moves in and out in a gentle rhythm deep inside your body.

Move your attention to your mind. Notice how your thoughts flow in and out, just like your breath.

Observe your thoughts without attachment or judgment, as though you were watching a movie. Feel peaceful in this awareness.

Realize that now you are no longer bound by time and space. This is your true nature — it has always been and will always be there. It expresses itself through the body and mind, but is not limited by them. Rest for a few moments in the stillness of that truth.

Concentrate again on your breath. Breathe a little deeper and, as you exhale, feel that you are bringing greater strength and energy into your body. Imagine this force moving out to every cell of your body — invigorating, nourishing and revitalizing your entire body.

Finally, slowly stretch out your fingers, toes, legs and arms. Take your time as you return to the full conscious awareness of your body. Feel that you are awakening from a deep sleep, renewed and alert.

Sit up slowly and remain in this powerful state of body and mind for at least one minute. During this time affirm to yourself that you will not let anyone or anything disturb you for the rest of the day.

****

Recommended Reading & Websites

Ulla Anneli's The Break™, relieve stress and

repetitive stress injuries with brief, easy-to-follow video exercise routines on your PC at home or work, **www.TakeTheBreak.com**

The New York Times Stress-Buster Crosswords: Light and Easy Puzzles, New York Times and Will Shortz, 2006, available on Amazon.com

Getting Things Done: The Art Of Stress-Free Productivity, David Allen, Penguin Group, 2001, available on Amazon.com

10 THE HEALING POWER OF LOVE AND SEX

"If you want to lead a peaceful, confrontation-free life, avoid talking about Sex, Religion and Politics!" For the most part, that's pretty good advice. Each subject is so complex, so personal and so sensitive, even in this day and age, that expressing one's views openly is like stepping into a minefield. So — in the interest of propriety, let's start with Love.

Love is the very best thing we do as humans. Some are better at expressing it than others but wherever love blooms, peace reigns. If you're a Babyboomer, you're at least 40 years old and, hopefully, you've had a lot of love in your life. If your fire of love is still burning brightly, that's a beautiful thing — and so are you!

On the other hand, if your fire of love has dwindled down to a few smoldering embers and your relationships are getting, shall we say, a bit chilly, I'd like to offer you a few thoughts and ideas that might help you "fan the flames."

If you're fortunate enough to have a long-lasting marriage or other loving relationship, you are blessed. To feel loved is to feel safe, supported and complete. To give love and receive it in return is one of Life's most beautiful experiences.

Life's routines, however, seem to use up all our time, energy and creativity. The regular, simple expression of our love and affection for our dear ones becomes infrequent or worse, inactive. The love is there and we know it but it has been relegated to the background.

Well, the good news is that this is easily remedied. Any one of the following things will open your arms and your hearts to each other and love will surge forth. You may be surprised at just how much.

1. Look into your dear one's eyes and say, "I love you." Simple, right? If it's so darn simple, why do so many of us forget to do it? Some people, most of whom are men, I'm afraid, find that simple expression to be embarrassing or even repulsive because they feel it somehow weakens them. Actually, the reverse is true. Those three words are incredibly empowering. Whatever your own situation may be, if you're not regularly expressing your love and admiration for your mate, you're missing out on something very important for both of you. Please don't let another day go by without saying these powerful and healing words.

2. Just like those "three little words", a hug that lasts five seconds or longer can bring love to the surface in a big way. Why? Because it's not casual and fleeting — it's sincere and lasting. It's comforting and reassuring. It feels good. Simple, right? Why don't we do it all the time, for Pete's sake? If touch has all but disappeared from your relationship, you're missing out on something special you both deserve. Please don't let another day go by without letting your dear ones feel your embrace.

3. Set aside a few hours on, let's say, a Saturday evening and take each other on a date. It might be dinner, a movie or anything fun you both like to do. Have your Date Night once a week and try not to let anybody or anything interfere with your special time together. Unrealistic, you say? I say if it's so easy to

fill the rest of your lives with busy routines, you can have at least one that's relaxing and pleasurable.

Allow these very basic ideas to trigger your imagination and creativity. Find your own unique ways to accomplish the same three things — private time for fun and pleasure, verbal expressions of love and loving touch.

What does love have to do with good health? Love is a positive emotion. Giving and receiving it does wonders for the body, mind and spirit. It stimulates your breath, your heart and circulation and it triggers hormonal flow, making you look and feel younger. Love lifts your spirit, lightens your step and makes you smile — and when you're smiling, people smile back.

So, nurture your loving nature. As exercise expands your muscles, expression expands your ability to love. Both are great for your health and well-being.

If Love is the cake, then Sex is the icing!

Have you noticed that when you reached 30, your birthday cards began to change? Suddenly, they were saying things like, "You know you're getting older when your birthday candles set off the smoke detector!" Then, when you're 40 and 50, your birthday cards seem to be more and more about your dwindling sex drive. The next thing you know, you're joking about it yourself, because in your case, it's true!

If you weren't much of a sensual or sexual person in your early years, or if you even found sex to be unseemly or even repulsive, then there's really not much to lose. You can't miss it if you never had it.

If you always had an exciting and fulfilling sex life, there's a great deal to lose. Fear and anxiety over this impending loss can be overwhelming. The drug companies capitalize on this fear by suggesting that their pill is the only way. Nothing could be further from the truth.

Granted, there are some conditions of mind and body that can interfere with your ability to perform normally and regularly. But many, many people attribute their dwindling sex drive to advancing age and they just give it up without a fight and they are just plain wrong!

If you believe that a healthy lifestyle can help ensure a long, healthy life, then you have to believe it can help you sustain a healthy sex life too, well into your 80's and beyond.

Allow me to make a few suggestions:

1. Develop and maintain a sexy attitude. There's a story about the 96 year-old man marrying a 22 year-old girl. His grandson says, "I'm worried, grandpa. I'm afraid the wedding night might be fatal." The old man shrugs and says, "Well, if she dies, she dies." See what I mean? Attitude!

2. Eliminate or change the things in your lifestyle that might be inhibiting your sex drive. Some prescription drugs for hypertension are better than others. Nicotine is a vasoconstrictor, which interferes with blood flow. Alcohol breaks down inhibition but

too much of it inhibits your libido. Stress does more to interfere with your sex life than almost anything else. Lovemaking is one of the most efficient ways of releasing stress.

3. Achieve and maintain a healthy weight in a healthy way. A well-nourished body is a sexy body, both in appearance and action. Exercise safely so that your muscles can tone and strengthen. Your goal is to be able to say, "You know, I look pretty damn good for my age!" By the way, weight loss is a wonderful by-product of lovemaking. Your metabolic rate increases, which burns calories.

4. If romance has always been in the forefront of your relationship, enhance it. If it has never been there, it's never too late to start. There's candle light, flowers, sensuous foods, music, dancing, hand-in-hand walks, backrubs and hot tubs. A getaway to a romantic spot might be an island in the Caribbean or breakfast in your own bed. Have you written any poetry lately? It's all up to you and your loved one. It's all about promoting closeness, touching, hugging and kissing. Romance is a form of foreplay.

But is sex good for your health? Oh yes, in so many ways.

Most people believe that, as we grow older, our desire for sex just naturally wanes. It's true that sex hormones are our master hormones and they affect every one of our body systems, including our moods, our creativity — even our looks. Sure, hormone deficiency affects us more as we reach our 50's and 60's. Women wrestle with menopause and all the physical and emotional turmoil it brings. Men just slow down, their libidos slip into neutral and, even though the thought of pursuing sex may arise, it's much easier to stay in the recliner.

We've inherited from previous generations the general belief that, after 60, it's just natural for sexual desire to recede. Don't fight the inevitable. Go quietly into that good night. Well, I'm here to tell you it doesn't have to be that way!

First, consider this: maybe it's not your sexual desire that's waning — maybe it's your loving feelings.

Take a moment to remember what it felt like to be happily, blissfully in love. Being in love is like taking a magic potion. People notice the change in you. They say you look better, younger, taller, happier and — more sexy. I've heard people say that they never felt more alive than when they were deeply in love.

Over the years, it's very likely that your comfortable familiarity with your spouse has overshadowed your feelings of love for each other. The love is still there and it's still a strong part of your bond, it just isn't being recognized and nurtured enough. Your daily routine may no longer have any time left for togetherness and intimacy. If this is true, and you don't have any major health issues, then you may be looking at the primary cause of your dwindling sex life.

People's relationships to love and sex are as individual as their fingerprints. And, sadly, there really is no universal piece of information that will give everyone a "Eureka!" moment. I suppose that's why there are so many advice and self-help books on the subject. So, I will offer some thoughts, ideas and suggestions that, hopefully, will stimulate your own thought, curiosity and creativity which will lead you to a renaissance of both your love life and your sex life.

Television ads try to convince you that sex-enhancing drugs are the answer. Not only that, they want to make you believe they are the easy, "quick-fix" for your problem. I'm very much against this "better living through chemistry" which seems to be pervading our whole society. Just reading the contraindications and interactions of the sex drugs should send a chill down your spine. Also, Hormone replacement and Human Growth Hormone raise the specter of cancer and are being studied thoroughly.

Get yourself a copy of the *Physician's Desk Reference,* which is available online and at most bookstores. Use it to investigate any medication you are taking now or in the future. Among all the potential side effects, I think you will be surprised at how many prescription drugs inhibit libido and sexual performance.

I advise people to consider these medications only as a last resort after lengthy discussion with your physician. Every single unnatural approach to renewing your youth and vitality comes with serious risks that you had better take a long, hard look at. I recommend you start with introspection to fully understand yourself and your needs. Then, as you make your changes, stress the *natura*l approach over the unnatural.

I'd like to give you a brief list of some of the most successful natural approaches to improving libido and performance for both men and women. Keep in mind that herbal products can also be dangerous if taken in large doses or in interaction with prescription medications. In some cases, they can be allergenic.

Chromium. Adult onset diabetes can interfere with sexual performance in men. According to *The Nutrition Report,* studies showed that supplementation with chromium helps balance and maintain blood sugar levels.

According to the Mayo Clinic:

Saw Palmetto may help men with the symptoms of enlarged prostate.

Black Cohosh may help women with symptoms of menopause.

DHEA may improve adrenal function, thereby improving the sex drive.

Also:

Progesterone cream, made from Mexican wild yam, is applied topically. For women it helps prevent vaginal dryness and vulvar dystrophy associated with age. For men over 55, daily use will help increase libido.

Ginkgo Biloba is one of the best-selling herbs in the United States. It can improve circulation in the brain, legs and, yes, the small arteries of the penis.

It also has been shown to improve a person's mental state by improving circulation in the brain. Now for a couple of "Don'ts":

Nicotine constricts blood vessels and inhibits orgasms, just in case you needed one more reason to quit smoking!

Alcohol is interesting because just the right amount is relaxing to the body and inhibition. But one drink too many begins to have a depressive effect on the body and mind. And, of course, when you're drunk, you're pretty much worthless in the sack. So, if you are having performance problems, check your alcohol consumption.

Speaking of natural approaches, the best place to begin is with some good old-fashioned introspection: that is, taking a good, close look at your mental, physical and spiritual self.

Let's start with these four things: Attitude, Appearance, Health, Fitness and Variety.

ATTITUDE

Check your attitude about love, romance and sex. Is it proactive or inactive? Is it forward-looking or living in the past? Are you giving it a go or just giving in?

What's your attitude toward your health and fitness? How about your energy? Are you energetic or are you thinking your "get-up-and-go" got up and went? Does your attitude need adjusting?

Your attitude is the springboard from which all your successes — and failures arise. If it's strong, positive and energetic, you're on the right path and you know it. If your attitude is fearful, negative and passive, you're on a downhill path and you don't want to go where it's leading. Change it!

Unfortunately, there's no attitude switch you can flip, no knob to turn. It's a mindset that have built for yourself with varying degrees of "help" from other people and events.. It can only be changed through thought and action.

Begin by saying to yourself, "This is how I am and this is how I want to be." Then plan the first step on your new path — and take that first step. Once you have taken action, you will find that all the subsequent steps will become increasingly easy. And, when people begin to notice your new attitude, and tell you about it, you'll be unstoppable!

APPEARANCE

So, how do you look these days? As the song goes, "Is your figure less than Greek"? Are you still hanging in there — or just letting it all hang out? What about your wardrobe? Is it Miami Beach in the 60's? Woodstock? Disco?

If you like what you see when you glance at the mirror or check out your reflection in a store window, great! If not, you're on the path to Frump City where the word "sexy" is not in the vocabulary!

When you're working on your new attitude, appearance is a good place to start. Look for new clothes, a new hairstyle, some color and style. Instead of watching the makeover shows on TV, give yourself one!

Believe me, when heads start turning as you pass by, you're going to love it!

HEALTH AND FITNESS

We've already discussed this but suffice it to say that good health and fitness do wonders for your attitude and your appearance. If you're on a fitness program, you know what I mean when I say you're "youthing." It's a great feeling and one you want to make the effort to maintain. If you're not on a program, please start one right away. At any age, movement always makes improvement.

VARIETY

Do you find yourself feeling bored, lethargic or just plain apathetic? You're probably suffering from what I call "Re-run Syndrome." By this I mean that your entire life has become a series of routines which repeat over and over and over. It's like watching the same TV program over and over.

"Re-run Syndrome" is one of the primary reasons that you may be suffering from bedroom fatigue or worse — you're dead in bed.

Well, for goodness sake, change the channel! Talk it over openly with your loved one. Don't be afraid of change, welcome it. Be creative. Be inventive.

Change the time and place for your romantic encounters. Take turns being the initiator. Be more impulsive. Dress sexy, act sexy, be sexy. Tease and please. Naughty can be nice, you know.

If you don't already know why they say, "Variety is the spice of Life," I'm sure you will!

Now I'd like to offer you some Yoga-based movements and techniques for couples which are designed to improve men's and women's capacities for love and sexuality.

BREATHING: Sit with your partner on the floor or the bed, facing each other, cross-legged, eyes closed, knees touching and holding hands. Do the Three Part Breath (Chapter 2, pp. 16, 17) for 3 to 5 minutes. In addition to the increased energy you receive, this technique creates a sensual effect and heightens your awareness. As you inhale, hold an image in your mind — such as the color red, a symbol of passion. Try to coordinate your breathing together. Inhale the last breath deeply and hold for at least a count of five. The exhalation of this last breath should be slow and complete. Open your eyes and look into each other's eyes for at least 10 seconds.

COBRA POSE: If you suffer from low back pain, I'm sure you know that sex is pretty much out of the question. In Yoga we say, "you are just as young or old as your spine is." The Cobra Pose is great for strengthening your lower back. Give it a try, being careful never to strain yourself and, if it works for you, do it often.

Beginning Version: Lie on your stomach, feet together, forehead on the floor, palms on each side of your head. Keeping your hands and forearms touching the floor, inhale and lift your upper body upward, looking up toward the ceiling with your eyes. Don't strain. Exhale as you turn your head to the left as if you are trying to see your heels. Return to the center, inhale, exhale turning your head to the right. Return to the center. Inhale, lower your head and rest, breathing normally. Repeat once or twice.

Intermediate version: Begin as before, this time with your palms on the floor, placed under your shoulders. First, using your back muscles, lift your upper body and your palms off the floor, feeling the entire weight of your upper body supported by your back muscles. Hold for a few seconds, then lower your palms to the floor and, keeping your elbows bent, push your upper body upward so the weight is supported equally by your lower back and arms. Don't strain. Breathe and turn your head left and right as before. Lower your upper body to the floor, breathe normally and rest. Repeat once or twice.

SIDE BEND: The side bend limbers your lower back, charges your adrenal glands and reduces your waistline

Sit cross-legged on the floor with a straight spine, your hands behind your head and your elbows pointing outward. Inhale deeply. As you exhale, bend to your left, pointing your left elbow toward the floor. Go as far as you can comfortably. Inhale and return to the upright position. Repeat, bending to your right side and return to the upright position. Inhale, exhale. inhale and repeat once or twice.

SIDE TWIST: Begin in the same position as the Side Bend. Inhale deeply. As you exhale, bend forward, pointing your right elbow toward your left knee. Go as far as you can comfortably. Inhale and return to the upright position. Repeat, this time pointing your left elbow toward your right knee. Don't strain. Return to the upright position. Inhale, exhale. Inhale and repeat once or twice.

HALF SPINAL TWIST: This is one of the most common poses in Yoga. It stimulates the ends of your spinal nerves and adrenal glands, rotates your spine making it more flexible and supple, induces energy and strength, reduces your waistline and improves digestion. It can be done on the floor or in a chair.

Floor Version: Sit with your knees bent to your chest. Extend your left leg out straight and cross your right leg over your left, foot on the floor. Extend your arms out in front of you. Inhale deeply. Exhale and twist to your right, placing your right palm on the floor behind you, close to your buttocks. Turn your head to look as far to the right as you can. Hold for a few seconds but don't strain. Inhale as you return to the center.

Now cross your left leg over your right leg, inhale and twist to your left, your left palm on the floor behind you close to you buttocks. Turn your head to the left. Hold a few seconds but don't strain. Inhale as you return to the center. Repeat once or twice on both sides.

Chair Version: (This version is perfect for the office, by the way.) Sit up straight in your chair, feet flat on the floor. Cross your right leg over your left and inhale deeply. Exhale and twist to your right, placing your right arm behind your chair and turning your head to the right. Hold a few seconds and inhale as you come back to the center.

Now cross your left leg over your right leg, inhale and twist to your left, placing your left arm behind your chair and turning your head to the left. Hold a few seconds but don't strain. Inhale as you return to the center. Repeat once or twice on both sides.

FORWARD BENDING: This is considered by many to be the best pose in Hatha Yoga. It massages the abdominal organs, stimulates the sex glands, and stretches the spine and hamstrings. Don't do this pose on a full stomach — please wait at least one and a half or two hours after a meal.

Sit on the floor with your legs stretched out. Inhale and raise your arms high over your head. Exhale and slowly bend forward as far as you can comfortably. Don't strain. Try to relax into the pose and hold as long as you can comfortably. Return to the upright position. Repeat once or twice.

If your back and hamstrings are very tight at first, you can place your back against the wall and bend forward. As an assist, you can put a towel around your feet and using your hands, pull your self forward and down. Please remember, don't strain.

These techniques and routines are beneficial in so many ways. I hope you will make them a part of every day. You'll feel better, look better and make love better!

* *

Recommended Reading & Websites

Too Tired To Keep Running, Too Scared To Stop: Change Your Beliefs, Change Your Life, Joyce Nelson Patenaude, Ph.D., Trafford, 2005, available on Trafford.com

The Proper Care And Feeding Of Marriage, Dr. Laura Schlesinger, HarperCollins, 2007, available on Amazon.com

Relationship Rescue, Phillip C. McGraw, Ph.D., Hyperion, 2000, available on Amazon.com

Sex Over 50, Joel Block, Ph.D. and Susan Crain Bakos, Reward Books, 1999, available on Amazon.com

2007 Physician's Desk Reference: Your Complete Print and Electronic Drug Information Solution, Thomson, 2006

11 MENOPAUSE — IT AIN'T FOR SISSIES!

What is menopause? Symbolically, for many, it's a sign of the end of youth and the beginning of old age. It's a change of life, it's a hormonal decline. For many women, it's accompanied by sleepless, sweaty nights, irritability, weight gain, depression, osteoporosis and lack of sexual desire. For most people, whatever it is, it sure ain't for sissies!

So how come some women sail smoothly through menopause and others suffer? First of all, some women are just simply fortunate and they barely have to give a thought to "the change." Others did their homework, informed and prepared themselves even before their perimenopause began.

In my case, I was going through a divorce, I had two teenage daughters in High School and I was under an enormous amount of emotional stress — talk about change of life!

But I was prepared. I knew that stress affects the hormones and glands, especially the adrenals. It was crucial for me to manage my stress as much as possible, so I increased my exercise, I kept my Yoga practice going strong and I read everything I could get my hands on about menopause.

I took lots of Vitamins A, B, C and E and Calcium, Magnesium, Boron, Flaxseed Oil and Omega 3. For hot flashes, I increased my intake of isoflavonoids, which act as a non-steroid estrogen. I adjusted my food intake to include Miso soup, Tofu, yams and lots of lentil soup and raw juices. For sleep, I took Melatonin and Valerian.

Many of my women friends had been taking Estrogen and Progesterone for long periods of time and some of them paid a high price — cancer — two of my dear friends died of breast cancer.

I decided to go drug-free and I had success with natural Progesterone cream as a means of replacing this decreasing hormone.

Then I started gaining weight around my waist and my favorite jeans were banished to the closet. Sit-ups didn't work and liposuction was out of the question for me. Then I discovered the insulin connection. Monitoring and controlling insulin levels helps control weight. Certain aspects of The Zone Diet were helpful to me too, particularly the negative effects of silent inflammation and high cortisol levels.

If you ask me, Life is precarious, Life is dangerous, and you deserve a pat on the back and a gold watch if you've made it through to menopause.

Each person experiences life events like childbirth from his/her individual perspective — there are lots of similarities and even more differences. Sometimes hearing about others' experiences can help give you a perspective on your own experience and how you react to it. So, with that in mind, allow me to offer two case histories.

VALERIE

"I come from a family of four sisters and, being the oldest, I was always the caretaker for my three younger siblings. My parents divorced when I was fourteen and my Mom got custody of all four of us kids and I never saw my father again. It was a terrible trauma for me and I have resented my father ever since.

"I left home after graduating from High School. I married my High School sweetheart and, about a year later, we had a son. It's hard to have a job, a marriage, a child and all the adult responsibilities, when you're still growing up yourselves. Our marriage only lasted for six years.

"If it was a struggle to survive before, now it went into high gear. I had a go at the movie industry, as an actress, God help me, and my son and I muddled through. All through this time I suffered from PMS and depression.

"I was about 42 and my son was a teenager when the first signs of perimenopause hit, with irregular periods, weight gain, insomnia and night sweats. It was miserable. My doctor put me on anti-depressants and hormone replacement therapy. To combat my bouts with panic, my doctor suggested I take deep breathing sessions and they were wonderful. At first I said, 'Who needs to learn to breathe, for Heaven's sake?' Well, I found out the answer is, 'Everybody!'

Conscious breathing techniques can be done anywhere to release stress. I still do them regularly.

"My menopause came early and violently. I felt I was losing my sexuality and I would never find love again. By now, I knew this was a process and, just like a very dark tunnel, I would eventually come out the other side. I continued my relaxation techniques, I put special emphasis on my spiritual study and, sure enough, six months later, I was better.

"I did marry again, this time to a much older man. You might say it was a 'marriage of convenience', but after the events of my previous two decades, convenience was looking pretty good! My husband is warm and generous and he has a great sense of humor. My son was off at college and I had lots of time, so I opened a successful antique business.

"I learned again that, just like a roller coaster, Life's twists, turns and bumps are much easier to take when you have someone to hold onto when the ride gets scary. This time of my life finds me much more happy and fulfilled than I was in my younger years.

TINA

"I have been very happily married to my husband, Sam, for over 30 years. We met in a dance class when we were both studying for our professional careers — he, a lawyer, and I, a teacher. We have two children, a boy and a girl, we live in a nice neighborhood, we've worked hard and enjoyed good health, except for my very bad PMS one to two days before my periods.

"At age 53, I started to have the first symptoms of perimenopause and they were strange. I was always the chilly one, you know, "Please close the window, honey, I'm freezing!" Suddenly, every night, the bottoms of my feet started burning like fire. It was weird. Before long I couldn't get to sleep without soaking my feet in very cold water. My periods became more and more irregular but, mysteriously, and happily, I no longer had my bouts with PMS.

"At 55, my periods stopped completely and my menopause began. I had always been such a good sleeper and I was very unhappy when my insomnia started. I had to get up at 6:00am on weekdays so I was usually in bed by 10:30 the night before. Here I was, tossing and turning, worrying about all sorts of things and trying to go to sleep. You can't TRY to go to sleep, you know. You either do it or you don't and most nights I didn't.

"The strange thing about my insomnia was that when it was at its worst, my busy brain and random, scattered thoughts would be accompanied by a song or sometimes two songs, words and all. It was all in my head, except for my husband's snoring. Some nights I could trick my brain by forcing it to calculate numbers, like how much money we would retire with at our present income level. I guess my brain would get bored or tired and just shut down and I could sleep. Other nights, nothing worked and I got to the point where I would just sigh and say, 'Oh well, here goes another sleepless night.'

"During this time, lack of sleep, combined with work and family stress issues, weakened my immune system. The result was frequent bladder infections, allergies and eczema. I started getting slightly anxious and panicky in stores and I was afraid it was going to develop into a full-blown phobia, or worse, agoraphobia. I literally gritted my teeth and gutted it out and the symptoms passed.

"I made a concerted effort to learn everything I could about menopause and attack it with all my guns blazing. Here's what worked for me. I added calcium-magnesium and vitamin D to my daily intake, along with fish oil, flaxseed oil and vitamin E. My moods began to stabilize very quickly and my general symptoms became much more manageable.

"I also put into daily practice what I learned in my Yoga class: conscious breathing, shoulder shrugs and neck rolls as quick pick-me-ups. This helped me so much in managing my daily stress.

"I realized that, with any difficult and momentous event in life, it's important to acknowledge what is happening, move forward and work on being happy. I'm determined to age energetically. What I mean by that is I want to resist settling in an easy chair, watching my TV and hoping to get vicarious pleasure from other peoples' experience. I want to create my own excitement through activities like music and seeing as much of the world as I can. My post-menopausal mindset is, 'Despite all the years I've lived, inside my deepest self I'm still only 35!'"

****

What most Boomers, men and women alike, have in common is the battle of the bulge. As much as two thirds of the population is significantly overweight, obese or borderline obese. No wonder type II diabetes is on a rapid rise.

I recommend you have your fasting blood sugar checked regularly. If you are pre-diabetic, you can reverse and even prevent this serious, life-altering disease by proper diet, exercise and weight control.

I did all these things and they really helped me weather the storm. Okay, maybe I didn't look like Suzanne Somers, but I sure felt more like the Ulla Anneli I've always been, with a strong sense of self and proud of my accomplishments.

I've been busy encouraging my Boomer students to follow this path or a similar one of their own design. Just as it's great to do exercise and weight control with a buddy, so it is with menopause. Find a menopause buddy and go through the experience together. The burden is always easier to bear when you have someone with whom you can share the load. When feelings of depression and anxiety set in, get out on the hiking trails, swim, dance — you'll be amazed how much control you can have over the process.

I threw myself into my work and found creativity I didn't know I had. I designed and co-produced two software products for stressed-out computer workers called "Ulla Anneli's The Break™" and "3 Minute Vacations™". I also produced a pilot video for women called "Menopause Buddies", which features especially designed exercise routines.

Okay, what about male menopause? Yes, there is such a thing. Contrary to popular belief, it's much more than buying a red sports car and chasing 20-somethings. It, too, is a hormonal decline which is accompanied by feelings of depression, loss of virility and vitality. The male physical symptoms are nowhere near as harsh as the woman's and they are more easily treatable with natural hormone therapy. The male psychological aspect can be equally difficult as the female one. I recommend couples counseling to help create an atmosphere of mutual understanding and support.

For most men, especially loving and caring ones, one of the most difficult periods in this stage of life is suffering through menopause with their mates. It takes a special measure of patience, caring and understanding. It takes a sense of humor, too. I've heard many couples say the journey was made easier by traveling the road hand-in-hand.

Is sexual intimacy important in a relationship? In some cases, the answer might be "no". There are couples who mutually agree that sex no longer plays an important part in their relationship but they continue to be good friends and partners.

If the answer is "yes" then, first, we should rule out medical conditions that can interfere with normal sexuality, such as thyroid problems, depression, diabetes, hypertension and side effects of certain medications.

Plan time for each other as you would for doctors' appointments. Create a sensuous environment free from any phone calls and avoid unromantic conversation topics like ailments and finances.

As our hormones decline, if we don't work on stimulating our desire for each other, our sexual desire will decline too. Sex shouldn't be a handshake, a routine duty to perform, but a wonderful union in a satisfactory relationship. Our sexual patterns, feelings and behaviors may change but the love and intimacy for each other can grow as we change.

Sex can be a reward for "good behavior" or it can be withheld as a form of punishment. Neither of these approaches is very healthy.

If you think about it, there's an irony here. Time was, it was a rare occasion when there was a little time, the kids were out playing, you two were alone and you made the best of your little intimacy window. Now, you've got nothing but time, the kids are out of the house permanently, you two are alone and intimacy doesn't even enter your minds!

Something is amiss here. If you're intimacy has

become infrequent or ritualistic, only on rainy Wednesdays before 8:00am, or the like, then you two ought to talk about how you can shake things up a bit. Then, for heaven's sake — do it!

Dress for sex. A menopausal woman who no longer finds herself sexually attractive or desirable may intentionally wear unattractive, baggy, rump-sprung sleepwear.

So ladies, get some sexy nightgowns, sexy sheets, look good, smell good and you'll begin to feel sexier. Buy your man some silk pajamas (he'll never buy 'em!). When your man looks good, tell him so.

So men: work on those flabby abs, dress better, look good, smell good, make little gestures and flatter your mate.

Tips and how-to's:

1. Find time, make time. Have a date night weekly.

2. Have candlelight dinners or champagne brunch in bed.

3. Make an extra effort to make birthdays and anniversaries special. Be romantic.

4. Talk about your fantasies together — you're too old to be shy!

5. Work on your fitness together — hiking, biking, swimming, workouts. As you see each other improving, it's exciting. If weight is an

issue, join Weight Watchers® together.

6. Do sensual things together, like massage, close dancing.

7. Shop together for new clothes. You'll have fun choosing new "looks" for each other.

8. Get a "nip and tuck" together. Don't overdo it.

9. If none of the above works, seek help, such as couple counseling, sex or relationship therapy like Imago therapy.

Menopause, male or female, isn't the end of your sex life (unless you want it to be!); it's a passage into a new phase of life. Let go of all those negative thoughts and emotions, most of which have been placed there by the media, not to mention those over 40 birthday cards.

You can put a new plan to work, a plan of your own mutual design. If your plan includes good nutrition, exercise, love and a positive outlook, your post-menopausal years can be your most fulfilling ones.

Instead of aging, think of yourself as "youthing"!

* *

Recommended Reading & Websites

The Wisdom of Menopause: Creating Physical and

Emotional Health and Healing During the Change, Christiane Northrup, M.D., Bantam, 2006, available on Amazon.com

The Pause: Positive Approaches to Premenopause and Menopause, Lonnie Barbach, Penguin Group, 2000, available on Amazon.com

12 PARENTING YOUR PARENTS

"There's no such thing as one-size-fits-all advice for people who are caring for their aging parents." So says Jane Wolf Waterman, LCSW, JD, a well known Beverly Hills psychotherapist. She continues, "The fact is that each individual situation is unique to each and every person involved. As therapists, we can help families improve their interpersonal relationships and cope with the day-to-day stress of care-giving. Beyond that, the best we can do is offer choices and resources and let families decide what's best for them."

Boomers who are caught in the middle between their aging parents and their teenage children still living at home are called "The Sandwich Generation." Some people are caring for their elderly parents, helping their twenty-something kids and babysitting the grandchildren — and many of those still work full time. I call these "The Double-Decker Sandwich Generation!"

Whatever your situation might be, the fact is that varying degrees of physical and emotional stress are constant companions as you go through this phase of life. Advance preparation, planning with special attention to caring for the caregiver(s), and using every resource available to you to its full advantage are the keys to your success.

If you are already caring for your aging parents or if you're fearful about what will happen when that time comes, I believe you will find the following case histories to be informative, helpful and encouraging.

ESTHER

"My Mom was a very dutiful and committed mother. She took care of us, she was always cooking meals — she was very loyal. She made sure we had our oatmeal in the morning, our lunch, and if we were sick, she took care of us. She was always there for us. She dressed me and my sisters in pretty, frilly clothes. She was not affectionate, just like her mother was with her, but she took care of us — that was her way. She was a great Mom but she was very much a disciplinarian.

"I also helped my mother with her Mom, cutting, grooming and coloring her hair. So at an early age I saw the pattern of taking care of your family and being loyal. I learned to pray from watching my grandmother. Little did I know how much that would help me when I was taking care of my Mom. My Mom was very young when her first symptoms appeared.

"It was Thanksgiving. I had made Kahlua and yams and we were all eating. All of a sudden, she started getting excited and standing up, talking loud. We all said, 'It's okay, Mom, it's okay.' At first I thought it was the Kahlua but later I realized it was the first of her erratic behavior. Another time a family member was sitting at the kitchen table with my Mom and he was petting the dog. Suddenly, she just turned and slapped him. We knew something was up. I guess my Mom knew something was up, too, because she had dented the car several times backing out to the street. She gave up driving by of her own volition, which was a huge saving grace for us.

"She was always a proud woman. She had worked her way up from poverty to being a top fur sales person at the May Company. She was very independent, but not very social. After my Dad died, she seemed to be doing pretty well on her own. My sisters and I would visit often and she seemed happy.

"One day I came to see her and she was telling me, 'You know your Dad was right, there IS a dragon that lives here and I saw him walking down the driveway when I was watering.' I spoke with my sisters and brothers and I heard a number of wild stories she had told them. That's when we decided to take Mom to the doctor. She was diagnosed with Alzheimer's and dementia and she was only about 65. It had a big impact on all of us. My mother was very upset because she had been healthy all her life. She didn't drink, she didn't smoke and she didn't take any medication.

"It's so sad to see her failing like that. Here's your Mom, who's always been so strong and now she's taking this downward turn without any hope of getting better. We had to decide very quickly who was going to live with Mom. My brother was just about to get married and his fiancée wanted to have her own family and they really didn't want the extra responsibility. About that time my job ended and we realized it was fortunate timing because, instead of paying people to take care of Mom, I could do it and Mom's Social Security payment helped with expenses.

"So I stepped up to the plate because I figured my husband and I had been through a lot and we knew how to roll with the punches. We wound up moving into Mom's home and dedicating ourselves to her care. It was tricky because we had to clean out some of her furniture to make room for ours. Because she was attached to her things as though they were treasure, we had to convince her we were buying her new furniture. Little did we know that this situation would last for almost four years.

"I took charge of her care but I always let her participate in cooking or house chores because she wanted to help and it made her feel useful. After a while, she could only manage little projects, like sweeping, cleaning the table or folding napkins. I thought it was right to give her a purpose for as long as possible. Dressing herself became more and more difficult. Blouses were inside out, zippers, buttons and snaps were left undone. She was becoming more and more like a child.

"Our social life was just about zero. The best we could do was to take an hour to go to Home Depot and get things for the house. That and my new garden were my escapes. When things got extra stressful, I would remember the breathing techniques I learned in Yoga and use them to relax. I had some resentment that I had to give up my life to take care of Mom. But then I remembered that she had taken such good care of me and my resentment turned back into to positive feelings, like loyalty, care, love and compassion. It takes a lot of positive energy and enthusiasm to keep a person like this going. I guess you could say I was my Mom's cheerleader.

"I managed for a long time but, as time went on, I knew in my spirit that it was getting to be too much for me. The financial situation was challenging. In the early days, I tried to work again part-time so we engaged IHSS (In-home Supportive Service) who sent a woman in to take care of Mom while I was working. Then I would take the next shift. It was exhausting, and finally, I had to give up my work and care for Mom full time again.

"I was able to use Mom's Social Security to take care of her, but it wasn't enough. I couldn't earn enough part time to make what we needed and I was beginning to feel stuck. I was starting to get weary, feeling stressed, emotionally drained and haggard inside. I was praying for my sanity. I knew it wouldn't be long before Mom couldn't walk any more. I realized that when I could no longer lift her, we would have to find a place for her.

"My sister found a place affiliated with Kaiser Permanente that would take Medicare/Medi-Cal and we talked to an attorney at In-home Solutions about the legal aspect. To get assistance, the person should have no assets. Everything should be transferred to other family members. He helped us take care of the details.

"Kaiser requires an Admissions Physical to evaluate her condition. They could see immediately that it was time for her to go.

"I dreaded that day. My brother and his wife helped me take Mom to the residence. I was so grateful because I could not have handled it alone. I had gotten so close to her. I guess it was easier for Mom. It was like she had become somebody else. She was compliant and cooperative. That part was easy."

"I hated leaving her there. When I got home, I missed her so much. There were so many emotions to sort through. After a while, it was like the stress was rolling off me. I had time again — for work, for play, for socializing, for laughter — for myself.

"I'm still watching over Mom, finding her the right chair, making sure they give her an afternoon nap — things like that. My brothers and sisters visit her regularly too, so it's okay.

"There's an image I have of my Mom not so long ago. She was pretty much out of it and it had been another stressful day. I was massaging her feet with lotion and she looked at me with clarity in her eyes and said, 'Thank you, my daughter.' I will carry that image with me always."

****

Esther's counsel to people is that you really don't know what you're getting into until you're in it, so the more you can plan ahead, the better.

1. If you can do so, set up a team so that no one person has to carry too much of the load.

2. Take care of all the financial details as soon as possible because they are sometimes too complicated to be accomplished quickly.

3. Early on, see if you can find an adult day care situation. Just like with young children, it helps to keep them busy and cared-for while you are working.

4. Maintain a social life for yourself. Have people

in for dinner if you can't go out.

5. Take frequent breaks and keep going with your crafts or hobbies.

6. Exercise. Exercise helps burn tension and anxiety. It oxygenates your body and it helps release endorphins, your "happy hormones".

7. Care-givers forget to pamper themselves. Take time to indulge yourself with baths, massages — anything that makes you feel good.

8. Avoid feelings of resentment. Stay in a loving place. This is difficult at times but remembering that they are much more like children than adults helps trigger your patience and compassion.

HEATHER

"Growing up in my parents' household wasn't the best it could be, to say the least. My mother was always complaining and crying about my behavior and my father was the punisher. Both were very good at being critical and not very good at being supportive, so I didn't grow up with a lot of self esteem. In later life, I would say our family dynamic could best be described as "mutually tolerant."

"I think I have a special situation because my mother's always been a child — I've been the adult — my mother never grew up. My father always took care of her and she's spoiled and quite demanding. On occasions, she can get downright mean and nasty. My father died a few years ago and my mother, who is 85 now, has gone downhill physically a great deal.

"We are fortunate to have the funds available to keep my mother in her home with attendants 24/7. The trouble is that she's become very frail, she's on a walker and she has started falling. Also, she's overweight because her only pleasure is eating and when she falls, it's very hard for the attendant to get her on her feet. She resists our attempts to get her into an Assisted Living place, saying she's not ready. I'm finding myself increasingly frustrated, irritated and impatient.

"My brother and I are hoping we can get our mother into the Jewish Home for the Aging, which is a great place because, unlike so many other places, if a resident's funds run out, they allow them to stay. My brother is the best son. He spends time with mother, pays bills and does what he can.

"A problem arose between my brother and me centered around the decline and death of our father. My brother, as the executor for our parents, decided to keep my father alive as long as possible. He had IV's, a tracheotomy, oxygen and a feeding tube. His eyes were open but it was like he was in a coma. I could not stand seeing him in that condition, so I either visited him for a few minutes at a time or I stayed away entirely. My brother resented me for that and it's carried over a little into our mother's situation.

"The sad truth is that my mother and I really don't like each other very much. My motivation as a care-giver doesn't come from a place of love, admiration or gratitude — it comes from my sense of duty. She's my mother and I'm duty-bound to take care of her. Doing the best I can for her is a statement about my integrity and character and I owe it to myself to do the right thing."

Heather's counsel:

"There are many organizations you can turn to for help and support. Food service, bath nurses and other help, both professional and volunteer is available to individuals and families. Research thoroughly, network with other people and really scope out what's available to you."

THE SISTERS

"We are so fortunate because our mom is not only cooperative in our efforts to care for her — she's an active participant! We developed the plan together. It was no problem getting her out of her home and into a wonderful independent living residence here in Los Angeles. Money is no problem because she has her own and is still managing it.

"This'll give you an idea of Mom's spirit. She met a nice man in the residence who's about six years older than she is. Before we knew it, they got married and moved in together! They're wonderful companions for each other. They hold hands and watch TV together and he plays the piano beautifully.

"We're also lucky that neither of us has to work for a living and we can devote a lot of time to Mom's needs, like shopping, doctor appointments and the like. She's been in the hospital a couple of times and we were able to spend lots of time with her and be sure she was getting the attention she needed.

"Our mom is a peaceful, easy, loving person. She was the typical 50's housewife with the high heels and the apron, waxing the floors — typical. We had lots of restrictions when we were kids. She forced us to go to church and we couldn't even go around the block on our bikes. Of course when we turned 18, we did everything — sex, drugs and rock-and-roll, which I guess is normal for over-sheltered kids. So here we are in this situation and we're doing everything we can for Mom because she did her best for us.

"One of our issues is that she's stubborn and she doesn't want to stay on her diet for type 2 diabetes. We're wrestling with this a bit because on one hand, we want to maintain her health as long as we can and on the other hand, at this stage of life maybe it's best to do what you want, eat what you want and take a lot of meds. She says, 'Eggs Benedict on Tuesday morning is my favorite meal and I want it.' When we take her out, she wants a burger or fried chicken and she really enjoys them. We want her to be happy but we don't want her to have a stroke or something that severely impairs her quality of life.

"We've both become medical advocates for Mom, which is really important. Recently, one of her doctors wanted her to have a surgery to correct a circulation problem which would have opened her leg from her groin to her ankle. We researched and found a surgeon at UCLA who did the same thing through a small hole in the groin. It was a huge difference in her recovery time. We respect doctors but we don't take their advice as gospel.

"The bottom line is we all know the risks and we all know where we're headed and we're all taking each day as it comes. In an odd and wonderful way, this is actually our best time of life with our mother."

The sisters' counsel:

1. Laughter. Keep them laughing. Keep your own sense of humor.

2. Keep them entertained. We use Netflix because they love old movies..

3. Do your best and don't feel guilty if you can't do something on a given day. You have your life too.

4. Teamwork. Share the load between as many people who are willing to take it. Communicate really well with each other.

5. Be patient. Don't get too emotionally connected to their fear and anxiety.

6. Take it one day at a time and one issue at a time.

7. Plan ahead! Don't delay until things really start to fall apart. Planning is good for their well-being and really great for your own peace of mind as time goes on.

PEGGY

"I come from a two-parent family but it wasn't close and it wasn't warm and fuzzy. My father was in the Army and the rest of us followed him around doing what we were told. My father died at 49 years of age. He was sent to Nagasaki two weeks after we dropped the bomb and he was in Korea when they were spraying Agent Orange. We believe this weird cancer he contracted was due in large part to his military service.

"My father's control over all of us was so strong that our relationships with each other were irrelevant. We were like individual units within his platoon. If we did something wrong we were in trouble with him. If mother tried to comfort us, she was in trouble with him. So everybody kept as low a profile as possible.

"Growing up, I was considered the black sheep of the family because I had a big mouth and no fear and I was brave and daring — and I was the one who caused the most trouble.

"So here Mom and I are. After my father died, my mother was always very independent and her independent spirit is still alive. I guess she could still live alone but she wouldn't be doing as well as she is. She really needs company and someone to keep track of her meds and such. She's really not very child-like yet but I do tuck her in every night. She uses a CPAP machine and she needs help going to bed. So I get her all set, tuck her blankets around her and say, 'Tuck, tuck — I love you.' She has pet names for me like cumquat, peapod and hibiscus — even poinsettia. It makes us laugh.

"Sunday is Mom's Day at my house. She never has to ask for it — it just is. On Sundays, Mom comes first. We do all sorts of things and we both look forward to it.

"Her main health issue is COPD, that's Chronic

Obstructive Pulmonary Disease. She developed Asthma in her late 30's, which is quite late. In those days, the basic treatment was to fill you with Prednisone and send you home, which wasn't very good for your future health. She suffers from anxiety and depression, for which she takes the usual medications, but she still wakes up almost every morning with intense anxiety. I believe this is due to too much or too little medication. She's starting to have gaps in her memory too.

"The great thing now is she still can keep herself busy. She loves the computer and she's on it all the time. She's a volunteer at the Senior Center and the Discovery Shop, where she and her peers talk over these same issues often, which helps us. What's not so great is she still drives her car once in a while.

"We've planned for the future financially. She has my house to live in, her medical care is covered — the rest we take as it comes, one day at a time. I have the name of very well-recommended nursing home so if she can't go on or I can't, we have a direction to go in. We sort of agree that if the time comes when she needs to be lifted and carried, that's something I can't manage and she'll have to go. Having that understanding is a blessing.

"As far as the rest of the family goes, I have a younger brother and sister. My sister lives in Missouri and my brother is here in California. They aren't in a position to contribute financially on a regular basis but in dire situations, they've helped. They're willing to let me take charge of Mom's care. I said, 'If you want in, let me know,' and they left it to me. My sister expresses her gratitude often but my brother and I have issues about my care-giving choices. He thinks I have control issues. When he communicated his feelings, I said to him, 'If you want to take over, I'll bring Mom over to your house this afternoon!' He declined. I feel bad about it, but I'm letting it go.

"Here's an interesting thing. I'm caring for my mother, yes, but I have to say that it has had a lot to do with changes in me: who I am and who I'm becoming. During this time that I've been exposed to all my mom's friends, I've discovered that I really love seniors. I've started a little business taking them to doctors' appointments or on shopping trips and other errands. After I retired I found my passion and my joy. My passion is Yoga and my joy is taking care of seniors. I combine the two by teaching Chair Yoga in Assisted Living places! It turns out that this journey is actually more about me than my mother. She's an important part of my self-realization.

"I know exactly when the essence of all this started. I saw a television news story about a woman caring for her mother, who was much worse off than my mother is now. She said how she was hating the experience and feeling anger and resentment toward her mother. Then one day this idea occurred to her, 'If it's this bad for me, how awful must it be for her? She has no choice.' This realization caused her to change her attitude completely. It helped me too."

Peggy's counsel:

1. Reach out to every resource available before you need them. Senior Centers are great because there are activities and lots of interaction with peers.

2. Support Groups, Support Groups, Support Groups!

3. Get equipment before you need it. If they're going to need walkers or scooters, get them early and keep them in the garage. When they need them, they're right there.

EVE

"My growing up was something out of "FATHER KNOWS BEST". Stay-at-home mom, my chemistry professor dad off to work Monday through Friday, you know. Dad had a temper but we had a really good relationship.

"Mom died of smoking-related brain cancer eight years ago and Dad lived alone in their 3-level townhouse for quite a while. He was coping and still quite busy but the place was just too big for him and the market was right so he sold it and moved into an apartment near me. He lived a pretty quiet life. He was still driving and he'd do his shopping, attend a senior group and an exercise class at the park.

"He moved two more times and we began to talk about him moving in with me. The problem was that my elderly mother-in-law was living in my guest room, where she had been for the previous eleven years — so you might say there was no room at the inn.

"She passed away about three years ago at age 102!" By that time, Dad had slowed down quite a bit. He stopped driving on his own and I was very grateful for that blessing. Also, I began to notice that very old, smelly food was in the refrigerator and he didn't seem to care, which was unusual. He was also becoming aware that his memory was beginning to fail.

"The doctors aren't sure if he's going into Alzheimer's or if he's having what they call TIA's, or Transient Ischemia Attacks. Another clue was he had a fall and hit his head and, quite a bit later, the doctors thought a mild stroke might have precipitated the fall. It was time for him to move in with me and I really wished we had done it sooner.

"Dad took part in making the financial arrangements. I have a power of attorney at his bank and I'm on the trust and he's fine with me handling everything. Dad's gotten pretty mellow in the last few years. He's much more easy-going, appreciative and it's making caring for him much easier. There's a Chinese proverb that says women get meaner with age and men get nicer. Maybe they're onto something!

"I was feeling a little guilty because I was working full time and he was spending a great deal of time alone. I found this wonderful combined adult and child daycare place called One Generation. I can drop him off in the morning and pick him up in the afternoon. They have food and activities and there are lots of people to talk to. At one point in the day, they let the kids mix with the seniors and it's fun for all. At his former senior center, if he got bored, he'd just walk home — five miles! At One Generation they don't let them out.

"We've had lots of drug issues. One memory

drug, Exelon, caused him to lose his appetite completely. He lost fifteen pounds really quickly. The doctor flipped when he saw my Dad and took him off the drug immediately. Dad's appetite came right back and he regained the weight he had lost.

"I want to keep Dad at home as long as possible. If he starts wandering and getting lost or if he no longer recognizes me or my daughters, I assume the next step will be to have someone with him all day. We did that with my stepmother for eleven years. You know it's interesting — the time my daughters and I had with my stepmother actually helped prepared all of us for this time with Dad."

Eve's counsel:

1. Be extra careful with medications. Read up on all the side effects and contraindications and how they react with other medications. Ask questions and if you see weird symptoms, make the meds a prime suspect.

2. Don't give your entire life to care-giving. It just doesn't work. Your health, well-being and peace of mind are just as important as your loved one's care. Take good care of yourself too.

PAUL

"I was born in Rio de Janeiro, Brazil. At the time my dad, who is French/Italian was working for the French Consulate there. My mother, who is French, was in charge of me and the household. When I was around two and a half, we moved back to France, where we lived until I was about eight and a half.

During this time, my sister was born in Versailles.

"Around this time we all moved to California where we already had a little colony of relatives — my grandmother, my aunt and two uncles. My dad was one of these handsome, daring risk-takers you hear about. He had been a fighter pilot in WW II and I guess that left him pretty fearless. He would try anything and if he fell on his face, he would pop right back up and try something else. Unfortunately, gambling was one of them.

"The problem was that he was usually in trouble to some degree or another and, finally, when I was about twenty, he left the family and went back to Europe. This was devastating to my mother who, for all his faults, was crazy about him. She never married again and she had only one serious relationship to which she couldn't commit. Part of it, I think, is that she had a very dramatic up and down life. She was born to a wealthy family and, coincidentally, her father left her mother too. During Word War II, her family lost everything and had to move around a lot. She was active in the French Resistance too.

"My Mom is a beautiful, emotional, loving, and devoted woman. She was wonderful with my sister and me and she has always been very close with my wife and our kids, whom she often took care of. She is a true artist and a very accomplished pianist and teacher. She's also quite opinionated, with a pretty much one-sided view of things. I'm a logical, A-to-B-to-C kind of thinker, while she is intuitive, and I've often found it difficult to reason with her. However, we were close in many other ways, such as love of music and nature and sharing a common sense of humor. I have always admired her ability to play some very complicated and difficult classical pieces.

"Mom's health problems started about twenty years ago with a degenerating hip, which ended up bone on bone. She was afraid of the surgery and endured great pain as she went from a cane to a walker and finally to her bed. About two and a half years ago, we moved her to our house and got a very nice lady to help her two to three times per week. Six months later, when the lady left our employ, my wife and I noticed that Mom was becoming quite dependent. A short time later, she was diagnosed with Alzheimer's and we knew we had to take action for her long-term care.

"The problem was that my wife, my sister and I were all working full time so we were left with two choices. One was to get more and more help for Mom and the other was to do it ourselves. We chose the latter and it all came down to me. Fortunately, I was financially able to take early retirement to care for Mom and that's what I did.

"When she finally consented to the hip surgery, a CAT scan revealed that being in bed for so long had caused her to develop blood clots in her legs. Before they could do the surgery, they had to put a filter in the Superior Vena Cava of her heart to keep clots from making their way around her body. The surgery was successful but her three week stint in rehab was a bust. She hated being bossed around and she was pretty uncooperative.

"She was doing okay for about four months post-op when a kidney problem almost took her life. She had always told us she had only one functioning kidney, which was true. What she didn't tell us was that the other one was never taken out. There it had been, festering inside her for decades, causing kidney and bladder infections. When her general health declined with age, so too did her immune system and WHAM!, she was hit by a near-fatal kidney infection and septicemia. It was touch-and-go for 48 hours but she survived.

"Mom became almost catatonic in the hospital, not reacting, not speaking — it was very scary. It turned out that when the doctors put her on this one very powerful antibiotic, they took her off her Welbutrin, an anti-depressant. I jumped on the internet and learned that a person can't stop Welbutrin 'cold-turkey' without having very severe symptoms of depression. Apparently, the doctors weren't aware of this. I was furious. They put her back on Webutrin and she began to come back.

"Being French/European, we don't even think about a rest home situation until it becomes absolutely necessary. Sure, there are such places in France but it's not a big industry like it is here. I guess it's a cultural factor.

"Mom's not able to walk now and we have her in a hospital bed, but she's pretty docile and easy to handle. I'm a big and pretty strong guy but I injured myself twice lifting Mom. The first was a tendon in my elbow and the second was my back. Since then, I've learned how to lift her without jeopardizing myself and it has been okay.

"Right now we can see that she is enjoying life and

that's an important factor. If my mother's mental state should prevent her from recognizing me and it no longer matters that it's me that's taking care of her, then I will put her in a nice place. At that point she'll need more medical attention and activities than I can provide and it will be better for her. Until then, I know she's happier at home."

Paul's counsel:

1. Make every effort to understand everything that is happening to your loved one, particularly what the doctors are doing. Don't be afraid to ask questions.

2. Protect yourself from physical and emotional stress. Take frequent breaks and do something you enjoy. In my case, it's long walks in the morning, reading, and playing the guitar.

3. Just as you did with your children, hire a "baby-sitter" and get out of the house. You might be amazed at how house-bound you can become in this situation.

MY STORY

"I was born on a farm in the central part of Finland. When I was only one and a half years old, my father died of wounds he suffered in the war between Finland and Russia. It was a terrible blow to my mother because she and my father were practically newlyweds with a baby daughter and here she was a widow at the tender age of twenty three.

"We were living in a big farmhouse in Pieksamaki,

Finland. My grandfather, my grandmother and my cousin Eine's mother were all parenting me. I never felt lonely on the farm. The farm was completely self-sustaining. We had meat, fish, dairy and vegetables, all fresh as they could be. It was hard work for the adults but it was a great place to be a kid.

"When I was about six, my mother decided to marry her second husband and we moved to an apartment in town. I was terribly sad because I missed the farm and my cousin Eine and I lost half of my mother's attention.

"About a year later, my mother gave birth to my half sister Aila. She was born without a thyroid gland and had many related health issues. My mother had even less time for me but it wasn't bad, because I always had clean clothes, and three really good meals on the table in a beautifully-kept household.

"My mother wasn't affectionate in the slightest way. She never hugged me and, to this day, she has never said she loves me. It was odd to have a distant relationship with my mother, but I didn't realize it until I visited friends' homes and saw what love and affection looked and felt like. Maybe that's why now I hug people, especially my two daughters, every chance I get!

"In my tenth year, something happened which literally changed the entire course of my life. A girl next to me in school was having trouble with a test and she asked me if I would help her. I did — and the teacher caught me. She stood me up in front of the class and humiliated me. When my mother learned about this, she beat me until I bled and she locked me in a dark closet for 24 hours. Later, for added punishment, I was sent away to an island to spend Christmas vacation with my aunt and uncle. It was a cold, dark winter — and I was miserable. The odd thing, which I didn't understand until much later, was that my mother kept yelling, not about what I had done at school but what I had done to her.

"My mother controlled pretty much every aspect of my life that she could. I wanted to be an entertainer or a journalist. She wanted me to be a nurse and off to nursing school I went. My nursing school was in Kuopio, Finland and I must admit that when I was finally out from under my mother's control, I went a little wild. About this time, I met a man from Bulgaria who had been my pen pal for five years and soon he was my husband-to-be. We were married in a civil ceremony and before too long, I left for the United States with my husband, never to live in Finland again. My mother was furious and my family was outraged — but I was free to live my life. I didn't even visit Finland for twelve years and for ten of those years my mother and I didn't speak.

"The first clue that my mother's health was declining was that she stopped riding her bike from the town to the cottage by the lake, a distance of some ten kilometers. Then, about eight years ago, I started getting letters from my sister Aila that mother was beginning to exhibit some uncharacteristic behavior. She was swearing, which she never did and she was verbally abusing Aila on a daily basis. She would sit alone and talk to herself for hours. Sometimes, for no apparent reason, she would break out in laughter.

"I felt frustrated because I couldn't help Aila and

worse, Aila couldn't help herself. Over the years, she always lived with mother; she never dated, much less married. Aila's thyroid deficiency caused her to have health problems and bouts of depression. She had become totally dependent on our mother and, despite all the unpleasantness building up around her, she could not bring herself to leave, even though she had the means to do so.

"In October, 2005, Aila passed away, a suicide, and my mother, at age eighty three, was alone for the first time in her life. Instead of reaching out to friends and relatives, she resigned herself to living in her own home until she dies, and she has stuck to her pledge even though she's had a couple of serious falls. She has also had a few dangerous mishaps with her medication, two of which resulted in hospitalization.

In 2006, when I was visiting, I learned from her doctors that she had been diagnosed with Alzheimer's *three years before,* and she never disclosed this to anyone.

"What's happening is that the same stubborn and independent spirit that got her through the loss of her beloved home in beautiful Karelia to the Russians, the uncertainty and poverty when she was a refugee and the loss of her new husband — that fierce pride is now her enemy.

"It's incredibly frustrating for me because she needs help desperately but she won't accept it from me or anyone. She won't even accept a Life Alert system. She should be handing over responsibility for her financial affairs to me, her only living child. I could force the issue but Finland's laws make financial and personal conservatorships very hard to accomplish.

"So, here I sit, 5,000 miles away, mostly helpless, waiting for that fateful phone call. I want to help my mother and bring some happiness to her final years but it appears I may never be allowed to do so. I send letters and photos which seem to cheer her up. She has stopped writing to me but we manage two or three telephone conversations per week. My cousin Eine and I have teamed together to send 3 home care nurses to attend to my mother. I visit for three weeks each year and do what I can. She still criticizes me mercilessly — but she loves my foot massages!

"It's hard to see her deteriorating mentally and physically. She is practically bed-ridden and she speaks often about dying and seeing my father in Heaven. The best I can do is to take care of my mother from this great distance and be ready for any circumstances, most of them dire.

"I am thankful for all the good things my mother did for me. I am proud of all her admirable qualities. When I'm with her, I hug her, I kiss her and I tell her I love her. When we are apart, I pray for her — and I have been able to learn to accept her as she is, not as I wish she could be."

* *

Recommended Reading & Websites

Caregiving As Your Parents Age, Dr. Linda Rhodes,

New American Library, 2005, available on Amazon.com

The Eldercare Handbook: Difficult Choices, Compassionate Solutions, Stella Henry, R.N. and Ann Convery, Collins, 2006, available on Amazon.com

Age Power: How the 21st Century Will Be Ruled by the New Old, Penguin/Putnam, 2000, available on Amazon.com

www.alz.org, The Alzheimer's Association, (800) 272-3900

www.aarp.org, American Association of Retired Persons, (888) 687-2277

www.caps4caregivers.org, Children of Aging Parents

www.eldercare.gov, Eldercare Locator Guide for finding community assistance. (800) 677-1116

www.caregiving.org, National Alliance for Care-giving

www.caremanager.org, National Association of Geriatric Care Managers

www. naela.com, National Academy of Elder Law Attorneys

www.ParentingOurParents.net Jane Wolf Waterman, LCSW, JD

13 NURTURING THE NURTURER

These case histories have one thing in common; care-giving is stressful and potentially hazardous to your health. If you're currently in a care-giving situation or you soon will be, I'd like to offer you some guidance that will help you keep your mental, physical and spiritual health intact.

Assemble your team

To the extent you can, assemble a team of family members to commit to regular schedules so the burden can be lighter for everyone. Loved ones who live in other parts of the country can do their share by making monthly contributions to a fund for their loved one's special needs.

Don't deny your denial

Perhaps most important, don't deny your denial. Be real about the facts of your care-giving experience and your ability to handle it. Support groups and therapy can help you with the difficult decisions. Guilt should never be a motivation.

Get your sleep

Make sure you're getting enough sleep; seven to eight hours are ideal. Nothing will wear you out faster than regular sleep deprivation.

Schedule stress breaks

Take time for yourself. Schedule stress breaks at least three times per day to "re-charge your batteries."

A stress break might be energetic, like exercise, or it might be restful, like a nap.

Exercise

Develop an exercise routine. Brisk walking is very good for all-around exercise. Hatha Yoga, with an emphasis on deep breathing, is a great stress reliever. If you can spare the time, I recommend two classes per week. If lifting is part of your care-giving, focus your exercise on stretching and strengthening your back.

Also, you can relieve the strain on your back with some of the products available for home care, such as back braces and slide boards for transferring from bed to chair and back.

Watch your weight

Work on keeping your weight under control. For many people, over-eating is a stress reliever, which is not good in situations in which stress is unrelenting. Ask yourself, "Am I eating because something's eating me?"

Try to co-ordinate when and what you eat with your schedule, so you can ensure peak energy when you need it.

Eat a good breakfast every day. Stay away from sweets, white flour, fast food and soft drinks. And, of course, smoking is dangerous to your health.

Family therapy

If depression is a problem, seek individual and group therapy. There are also many support groups designed specifically for care-givers.

Vary your routine

If your routine gets boring, please change it. Plan activities that are stimulating, because variety and excitement really help combat depression. Try to avoid the hospital atmosphere. Add aromatherapy, music, flowers and funny movies.

Delegate responsibility

To every extent you can, delegate errands to relatives, friends or volunteers. Saving your time saves your energy.

Getaways and date nights

It's important for care-givers and their spouses, family or friends to get away for an evening or a "date night" or, even better, a weekend. The military advocates R & R, (Rest and Recuperation) and so should you! Spontaneity is difficult in home care situations, so plan ahead. It's great to have something to look forward to.

Keep in mind that the quantity and quality of your care-giving relates directly to the degree you're able to take care of yourself.

* *

Recommended Reading & Websites

The Empty Nest: 31 Parents Tell The Truth about Relationships, Love and Freedom After The Kids Fly The Coop, Karen Stabiner, Hyperion 2007, available on Amazon.com

The Road Less Traveled, 25th Anniversary Edition: A New Psychology Of Love, Traditional Values and Spritual Growth, Touchstone/Simon & Schuster, 2003, available on Amazon.com

The AARP Guide To Pills: Essential Information On More Than 1,200 Prescription Medications, Including Generics, Side Effects and Drug Interactions, Maryanne Hochadel, PharmD, BCPS, Jerry Avorn and Bill Thomas, AARP/Sterling, 2007, available on Amazon.com

14 RANDOM THOUGHTS & REFLECTIONS

Life is breath — breath is Life. All of us, and every person who has ever lived, have one thing in common. We came to this world with an inhalation and we will leave it with an exhalation. We must make the most of all the breaths in-between.

This poem is all about making the most of it:

THE DASH
by
LINDA ELLIS

I read of a man who stood to speak
At the funeral of a friend.
He referred to the dates on her tombstone
From the beginning to the end.

He noted that first came the date of her birth
And spoke the following date with tears,
But he said what mattered most of all
Was the dash between those years.

For that dash represents all the time
That she spent alive on earth.
And now only those who loved her
Know what that little line is worth.

For it matters not how much we own;
The cars, the house, the cash.
What matters is how we live and love
And how we spend our dash.

So think about this long and hard:
Are there things you'd like to change?

For you never know how much time is left
That can still be re-arranged.

If we could just slow down enough
To consider what's true and real
And always try to understand
The way other people feel

And be less quick to anger
And show appreciation more
And love the people in our lives
Like we've never loved before.

If we treat each other with respect
And more often wear a smile
Remembering that this special dash
Might only last a little while

So when your eulogy is being read
With your life's actions to re-hash
Would you be proud of the things they say
About how you spent your dash?

* * * * * * * * * * * * * * * * * *

Don't let go of your inner sense of child-like wonder and your own magnificence. When you see something new and beautiful, take it into the deepest part of yourself and react from there. I call it "The Inner Wow!"

* * * * * * * * * * * * * * * * * *

Life is a journey of deep, dark valleys and high, bright mountains. Even the darkest valley serves a purpose for our inner growth. Without it, how can we fully appreciate all the good in our lives?

****

If you know how to worry, you know how to meditate. Worrying takes the same time and the same focus of the mind. Why not meditate instead? Instead of littering your mind with unhappy thoughts and negative fantasies, why not spend the same time emptying your mind of all negativity and finding your peace within?

****

Do you sometimes ask yourself:

Did I reach my highest dreams or did I settle for mediocrity? Am I fulfilling my deeper purpose on earth?

Have I touched people's lives in a meaningful way and made a difference in the world?

Did you marry your high school sweetheart and live happily ever after? Did you marry a stranger and remain in an unhappy relationship? Did you divorce?

Did life go by painfully fast: going to school, getting a degree, getting married, raising kids, maintaining relationships, paying bills, and you're wondering, "Is that all there is?" Is there a deeper purpose and meaning behind all this?

Whatever your spiritual beliefs may be, we all have a longing deep down inside of us to find our

Divine Self, to feel at home and safe, and to feel that our souls are resting and at peace.

Even when things all around us are chaotic, we can trust that God has a plan for our lives at any state, giving assurance that our lives are unfolding as they should.

* * * * * * * * * * * * * * * * *

Fear and faith cannot exist together at the same time. Faith is the antidote for fear.

Here's what Nelson Mandela said about fear in his inaugural speech in 1994:

"Our deepest fear is not that we are inadequate. Our deepest fear is that we are powerful beyond measure. It is our light, not our darkness, that most frightens us. We ask ourselves, 'Who am I to be brilliant, gorgeous, talented and fabulous?

"Actually, who are you not to be? You are a child of God. Your playing small does not serve the world. There is nothing enlightened about shrinking, so that other people won't feel insecure around you.

"We are born to make manifest the glory of God that is within us. It is not just in some of us; it is in everyone. And, as we let our light shine, we unconsciously give other people permission to do the same.

"As we are liberated from our own fears, our presence automatically liberates others."

If fear weakens us and makes us ill, faith strengthens us and heals us. Hopefully, we are on the right path and the road signs lead us to our destination.

Through faith and prayer we can celebrate life and move on to our "Golden Years" with grace and courage. Regardless of our age, we can acknowledge the Divine Child that dwells within us.

* * * * * * * * * * * * * * * * * *

It is time to take inventory of our lives and come in peace to ourselves and others — to forgive and move on with grace and an attitude of gratitude.

* * * * * * * * * * * * * * * * * *

Life is the only teacher that gives the tests first and the lessons afterward. Life's lessons are needed for our inner growth.

Even our enemies have been our teachers.

* * * * * * * * * * * * * * * * * *

Even though you've had disappointments, broken relationships and dreams, ask yourself what you have given to life and what has life returned to you.

Don't give up on your miracles. Have an expectancy that all is well with you and with your loved ones, far or near, and you are enjoying each day in a wonderful way.

Repeat this twice every morning when you wake

up: "All is well — now and always." It's a tiny but powerful meditation to help dispel fear and keep your mind on the right track.

* * * * * * * * * * * * * * * * *

You have made a difference in other people's lives and now is the time to make a difference in your own. Let your inner messenger guide you even deeper within as the years go by. So, if you've lived to be 60, take extra good care of your physical, mental and spiritual self and you can look forward to many more years of inner reflection and the joy of giving and receiving love. The best is truly yet to come.

* *

Recommended Reading & Websites

God Is No Laughing Matter, Julia Cameron, Penguin/Putnam, 2001, available on Amazon.com

The Transparent Life, Naomi Judd, J. Countryman, 2005, available on Amazon.com

Spiraling Through the School Of Life: A Mental, Physical and Spiritual Discovery, Diane Ladd, Hay House, Inc., 2006, 2007, available on Amazon.com

15 YOUR GOALS ARE YOUR VISION

Every New Year we make resolutions, which we usually forget as early as February. We really do want to make changes in our lives and habits but we seldom think about what it will take to accomplish them.

Let me offer you a little worksheet where you can write some notes on your personal goals, which create your vision for the future. Give the process some serious thought and write your goals in these lines.

What are your health goals for five years from now?

____

____

____

____

____

____

What about your weight?

____

____

____

____

____

Now, where do you want your relationships to be in five years?

____

____

____

____

____

____

How's your social life? What improvements would you like to make?

____

____

____

____

How can you improve your financial affairs?

Do you need to advance your spiritual growth? If so, what changes would you like to make?

Do you have enough time for your favorite hobbies? If not, what do you love to do and how can you make the time?

____

____

____

____

____

Do you love to travel? Where would you like to go in the next five years?

____

____

____

____

____

____

****

Keep these goals somewhere where you can revisit them regularly. They will gently remind you about where you want your life to go.

* *

Recommended Reading & Websites

Your Best Life Now: 7 Steps For Living At Your Full Potential, Joel Osteen, Faith Words, 2004, available on Amazon.com

The Purpose Driven Life: What On Earth Am I Here For?, Rick Warren, Zondervan, 2002, available on Amazon.com

The Power Of Now: A Guide To Spiritual Enlightenment, Eckhart Tolle, New World Library, 1999, available on Amazon.com

INDEX

W

Y

Z

www.ingramcontent.com/pod-product-compliance
Ingram Content Group UK Ltd.
Pitfield, Milton Keynes, MK11 3LW, UK
UKHW020141250726
13967UKWH00002B/801

9 781425 117122